50 Human Studies

In Utero, Conducted in Modern China

Indicate Extreme Risk

~for~

Prenatal Ultrasound

A New Bibliography

Commentary

by

Jim West

© 2015 harvoa
All rights reserved.
ISBN 978-1-941719-03-9
Library of Congress Control Number: 2015944054

Publisher's Cataloging-in-Publication Data

West, Jim, 1947-
50 human studies in utero, conducted in modern China,
indicate extreme risk for prenatal ultrasound:
a new bibliography / Jim West.
pages cm
Includes bibliographical references.
ISBN: 978-1-941719-02-2 (pbk, color)
ISBN: 978-1-941719-03-9 (pbk. b/w)
ISBN: 978-1-941719-01-5 (e-book, color)
1. Ultrasonics in obstetrics. 2. Ultrasonic imaging.
3. Medicine—Research. I. Title.
RG527.5.U48 W47 2015
618.207543—dc23   2015944054

Understatement

"It must surely be unwise to... await conclusive evidence of harm before being cautious about the use of ultrasonography."

"A Review of Potential Adverse Effects of Antenatal Ultrasonography",

by A. J. Baczkowski, Dept. of Statistics, Univ. of Leeds, Dec. 1997

Contents

Preliminary Notes

Disclaimer: Those seeking medical advice should consult medical professionals. The reader should discuss this work with professionals to clarify and verify issues herein. The author is not an authority, and thus, his findings may not reflect current practice, knowledge, or state of the art.

This book represents views acquired by carefully accepting the results of critical ultrasound studies that have been ignored, overlooked, or dismissed. These are the Western animal studies exemplified by Liebeskind (1979-1981), Anderson and Barrett (1979-1981), Ang (2006), Ellisman (1987), Saad and Williams (1982), and the Chinese Human Studies.

This book is intended to encourage reasonable discussion of the contradictions that range throughout the history of medical and therapeutic ultrasound. Currently there does not appear to be a sufficient authoritative public forum for discussion and evaluation of these contradictions.

Any views derived from this book are inconclusive pending authoritative review.

Even if authorities were to lend weight to this book's message (that ultrasound is hazardous), the application of that message to any specific human case could still be questionable due to the complexities of exposure, human biological responses, and specific case requirements.

This book is not written in stone. It should be challenged and if found in error, corrected, the results of which will be included in future publications and/or www.harvoa.org.

Several scientists have engaged the author in discussion on various topics. They did not request confidentiality, but nonetheless, they remain anonymous due to the sensitivity of the topic.

Editorial assistance: Claus Jensen, Ruth Parnell, and others.

Acknowledgement: Anthony Brink, Mitchel Cohen and the No Spray Coalition[172], Trelane Freeman, Diane Gregg, Tedd Koran, Barbara Kovacs, Ramiel Nagel, Gary Krasner, Sheri Nakken, The Perth Group, Jon Rappoport, Chris Rawlins, June Segal, Eugene Semons, John Scudamore, Matthias Weiser, and others.

A small technical glossary is provided.

Annotation is placed in [brackets]. Emphasis is **bolded and *italicized***.

Join the email list at harvoa.org for notifications of new material, corrections, and updates.

Praise for this book

Since publication in 2013, there has been no negative commentary; there have been no challenges to this book. There is much acclaim, for example:

Jon Rappoport, Investigative Journalist

> *The great Jim West has done it! His meticulous analysis has turned the establishment on its head. If I were the king of Pulitzers, I would give him a dozen. He is what truly deep reporting is all about.*

Eitan Kimmel, PhD, Dept of Biomedical Engineering, Technion Institute, one of the world's premier research centers.

> *Your book is wonderful. You found the human studies. Chapter five is terrifying! I wish I were wrong.*

Sam Milham, MD, MPH, former epidemiologist for New York State, professor, author, and pioneering EMF scientist. sammilham.com

> *Great job. Your book is doing a valuable service to the childbearing public... You just cannot expose a fetus to this much energy without doing harm. For example, see Newnham (1993).*

Zvonko Hočevar, LLT Dr, Ljubljana University Medical Centre

> *Congratulations for your book and your courage in presenting this topic to public. Heartfelt thanks! I did my Doctorate of Science, finding 'no evidence based medicine' supporting 'safety' of ultrasound in IVF (in vitro fertilization) procedures.*

Manuel F. Casanova, MD, Vice Chair for Research in the Department of Psychiatry and Behavioral Sciences at University of Louisville.

Dr. Casanova is a prominent neuroscientist, with groundbreaking research in the field of cortical neurocircuitry, e.g., brain minicolumns.

> *This is important work. Attention must be brought upon the subject. Ultrasound is more than taking pretty pictures of babies. We are learning about side effects and mechanisms of potential harms that have not been the object of safety studies, least regulations. You have brought together the field by summarizing many different areas that bear on the subject, from physics to biology and medicine. Your writing should raise awareness in the layperson, that ultrasound is a "buyers beware" market. That before the glacial pace of our government moves to take action it is their responsibility to become informed and take adequate decisions.*

William O'Brien, Jr, PhD, prominent ultrasound scientist, author, former President of AIUM (American Institute of Ultrasound in Medicine), former Chair of AIUM Bioeffects Committee, and Director of Bioacoustics Research Laboratory.

O'Brien authored a commentary of JZhang (2002) in response to my lobbying. Extract:

> *The study, JZhang (2002) was relatively well done and documented with a dose-effect response... The study needs to be reproduced... 13 mW/cm2 is really low... The finding is important... the SPTA [intensity] levels do not support [the thermal] view [i.e., a nonthermal mechanism is supported].*

Stephanie Seneff, PhD, Senior Research Scientist, MIT

I read your book and I was fascinated by it! ...ultra-sound as a possible danger during pregnancy... I am now much more aware.

Tedd Koren, DC, korenpublications.com

Thanks so much. I can always depend on you for great info. You are a true seeker of truth.

Kelly Brogan, MD, KellyBroganMD.com

Human studies condemn ultrasound! Jim West has compiled the largest bibliography of human ultra-sound studies.

Gary Krasner, Coalition for Informed Choice

Jim West is the leading independent researcher of disease causation from chemical exposure. Now he has written a ground-breaking book that documents the inconvenient facts about the dangers of ultra-sound. Parents and medical professionals should re-consider the cost/benefit of ultrasound.

Ramiel Nagel, author of Healing Our Children

There is clear evidence that ultrasounds during preg-nancy can change fetal tissues. Jim West dug up this impossible to find evidence to make it obviously clear that we should not be haphazardly using video ultra-sounds when less invasive technologies can be used.

Amy Worthington, wi-cancer.info

I have read this book slowly and every page is marked, underlined and highlighted. It is brilliant the way it ties together so many loose strings and exposes the lies. In my opinion, this book is THE most important work of our times.

Nexus Magazine

Western scientific and medical professionals do not seem to be aware of the many human studies that have been conducted in China which clearly indicate damage from the use of diagnostic ultrasound. It is time that they examined this new compilation of research.

Russell B. Olinsky, M.S. Environmental Specialist

Jim West should get a Goethe Prize.... The ramifications should be huge, but alas I do not' expect change due to vested interests.

Daniel Maciejewskion

This is a well written book on a crucially important subject... Even before reading this book, I was convinced that prenatal ultrasound is leading to the boom in autism and other developmental disorders in children. After reading this book, any doubt I had about the damaging effects of ultrasound are gone. Jim West does a wonderful job of not only presenting the research, but providing a framework for understanding what is going on.

Michael Ellner, HEAL-NY

Jim West's passion and skill for finding, checking, exposing bogus medical facts and the economic, political, and social forces that drive and protect conventional medical practice is legendary among alternative health care activists.

1 | The Chinese Human Studies

This book presents a new ultrasound bibliography, i.e., the Chinese Human Studies (CHS). Prior to this publication, with few exceptions, these studies have not been acknowledged within the Western realm.

The CHS are modern clinical studies, with analytic technology generally beyond the tradition of Western ultrasound science. The CHS were conducted during a virtual explosion of ultrasound research in China, 1988-2011. They investigate damage to the human fetus in terms of causation by diagnostic ultrasound (DUS). They support and reference critical Western animal and cell studies that had been neutralized, ignored, or denied funding for continuation.

The CHS method: Women who have elected to have abortions are exposed to diagnostic ultrasound before the abortion. The abortive matter, such as, the brain, kidney, eye, or chorioamnion tissue, is examined in the laboratory via biochemical analyses and/or electron microscopy.

Western authorities claim DUS is harmless, based upon their contention that there are no human studies to confirm hazards that have already been found in some animal and cell studies.

An authoritative review, submitted to the *Journal of Ultrasound*, by the "United States Marine Corp and the U.S. FDA", provides assurance.

> "Although laboratory studies have shown that diagnostic levels of ultrasound can produce physical effects in tissue, ***there is no evidence from human studies*** of a causal relationship between diagnostic ultrasound exposure during pregnancy and adverse biological effects to the fetus."[32]

Douglas L. Miller, PhD, describes the authoritative beginnings of safety assurance.

> "Safety assurance for diagnostic ultrasound in obstetrics began with a tacit assumption of safety allowed by a federal law..."

The CHS contradict the safety aspects of those statements of assurance.

With the CHS, this book supports established critical positions by arguing DUS causation or initiation for Autism Spectrum Disorder (ASD), ADHD, personality anomalies, ophthalmological diseases, various malformations, skin diseases, and allergies.

While DUS causation can be argued in isolation, there is the very real and practical concept of toxic synergy. It should be argued that DUS initiates vulnerabilities to secondary stressors such as vaccines or other pharmaceuticals. This conforms with the views of some mothers who record every detail of their child's birth and development, and see their children autistic at birth or triggered autistic by vaccines or other pharmaceuticals. This concept, as a causation theory, is supported by ultrasound synergy studies such as Qian (1996).[36]

Novel DUS causation models will be introduced here, and detailed in a forthcoming publication. Examples:

1) Chorioamnionitis, a common prenatal disease, an inflammation of the chorioamnion, the maternal-fetal junction, the maternal protection of the fetus.

2) Jaundice, a common neonatal disease.

3) Childhood cancers, e.g., leukemia, lymphoma, brain cancer, etc.

2 | CHS Example Image

The CHS are usually published in Chinese language. Some have added English summaries, no more than the title and abstract. These studies can be translated with online software and edited to make them more presentable. Fee-based translations are also an option from the source databases. Editing requires some familiarity with ultrasound terminology.

See below, a CHS example, imaged, the first page of Zhiyou Zhang (1994), "Study On The Effect Of Newborn Erythrocyte Immune Function Exposed To Diagnostic Ultrasonic Irradiation In Pregnant Women". The study demonstrates that the fetus/infant Red Blood Cell (RBC) immune system is compromised by DUS. This study is discussed in Chapter 5.

See the original image. [Image→]

120　　　　　　　　　　　　　　　　中华超声影像学杂志 1995 年 5 月第 4 卷第 3 期

诊断用 B 型超声对胚胎绒毛组织的影响

韩秀丽　郭宏伟　聂　伟　李桂芹　范晓红

　　摘　要　经腹对 40 例宫内胚胎绒毛组织进行不同时间辐照后,获得其超声下宫内妊娠囊大体形态变化及光、电镜下绒毛超微结构变化.结果发现:超声下观察持续辐照首先可见妊娠囊收缩,绒毛板呈细锯齿状,变厚,回声偏高,之后妊娠囊与宫壁间可见无回声带,囊壁毛糙,胎芽轻微蠕动,胎心节律变化. A 组(照射 5 分钟)病理组织学变化不明显.B、C、D 组(照射 10、20、30 分钟)绒毛上皮细胞出现不同程度损坏,胞体大,水肿,变性,坏死,核固缩,疏电子性.病理组织的变化程度说明了超声辐照时间越长,其组织破坏程度越显著.早期妊娠保留者,应适当充盈膀胱,尽可能一次完成不可以短时间内反复辐照.在观察某一固定区域时一次连续辐照时间应限于 1 分钟为妥,完成全部操作限于 5 分钟以内.
　　关键词　超声剂量　绒毛组织　妊娠囊　光镜技术　电镜技术

Effect of Diagnostic B—ultrasound on the Embryo Villi Tissuses
Han Xiuli,Guo Hongwei, Nie Wei,et al
Gyneclogic and Obsteric Hospital of Mudanjiang,Mudanjiang 157000
　　Abstract　Under the different time of ultrasonic examination the ultrastructure of the pregnant cyst and villi tissues of 40 cases of embryo were studied. We have found that the longer time of the B—ultrasound examines, the more obvious of the villi tissues change. The change of group A within 5 minutes radiation is not obvious. The villi epithelium cells of group B, C and D for 10, 20 and 30 minutes radiation are swelling, degenerating and necrotic. So we should inform that the woman who continues pregnacy would be full of their bladders and the time of ultrasonic examination would be short, avoiding repeated radiation. It is very safe that the B—ultrasound examination lasted for 5 minutes and the observation for a fixed area would be limited within 1 minute.
　　Key words ultrasonic dosage　villi tissuses　pregnant cyst　technique of electron microscope

　　超声对胚胎早期安全的影响被国内外超声界所重视[1].我们经腹对宫内胚胎组织绒毛组织进行不同时间辐照,以获得其超声下宫内妊娠囊大体形态变化及光、电镜下绒毛超微结构变化及较安全时间范围进行研究.

资料和方法

一、病例来源

　　研究对象为 1993 年 12 月~1994 年 2 月宫内妊娠 45 天~55 天的孕妇,自愿终止妊娠者.无服药、X 线接触或遗传病史,无阴道流血.对照组妊娠期无 B 超接触史.共 50 例.

二、方法

　　1.超声诊断仪:Aloka~620 型,探头频率 3.5MHz,将研究对象随机分 5 组,每组 10 例, A 组辐照 5 分钟,B 组辐照 10 分钟,C 组辐照 20 分钟,D 组辐照 30 分钟,E 组为对照组.经腹部按不同时间垂直妊娠囊持续辐照,同时观察其妊娠囊及周围组织形态变化,观察中用 SONY—UP—850 型摄片记录.10 小时内终止妊娠,留取标本送病检.

　　2.50 例绒毛组织标本均以 10%福尔马林固定,石蜡包埋,HE 染色,光镜观察.

　　3.电镜技术:10 例标本(不随意)从每组中

作者单位:157000　牡丹江市妇产医院

3 | Fundamentals

There are three levels of DUS knowledge.

1) Western medical authorities loudly proclaim to the public, "Ultrasound is harmless", and, "Fetal ultrasound has no known risks".

2) Most scientific authorities qualify those claims quietly, publicly, but not in mainstream media. They conclude that ultrasound is apparently safe, while recommending further study.

3) A small minority of professionals and independent researchers are unapologetically critical. I quote four.

Dr Mendelsohn was the Chairman of the Hospital Licensing Committee of the State of Illinois, and former National Director of Project Head Start's Medical Consultation Service.[9]

> "Ultrasound is the latest example of an unproven technology being sold to the public as being 'perfectly safe.' It falls in the same class as painting radium on watches, fluoroscoping children's feet in shoe stores, routine mammography, routine chest X-rays, radiation therapy for tonsils, exposing army personnel to atomic bomb tests - in each case, the medical profession failed to take the necessary steps to protect people against a malignant technology whose risks were already well understood."[7]

Marsden Wagner, for 15 years, former Director of Women's and Children's Health in the World Health Organization:

> "Although we now have sufficient scientific data to be able to say that routine prenatal ultrasound scanning has no effectiveness and may very well carry risks, it

would be naive to think that routine use will not continue. Unfortunately, medical doctors are inadequately educated in the basics of scientific method. It will be a struggle to close the gap between this new scientific data and clinical practice."[10]

Caroline Rodgers, author and researcher, refers to Grether (2009), a large population study:

> "Particularly confounding is the fact that ASD plagues the children of high-income, well-educated families who have the best obstetrical care money can buy. Why would women who took their prenatal vitamins, observed healthy diets, refrained from smoking or drinking and attended all regularly scheduled prenatal visits bear children with profound neurologically based problems?"[11]

Sarah Buckley, MD:

> "Although ultrasound may sometimes be useful when specific problems are suspected, my conclusion is that it is at best ineffective and at worse dangerous when used as a 'screening tool' for every pregnant woman and her baby. [...] Treating the baby as a separate being, ultrasound artificially splits mother from baby well before this is a physiological or psychic reality. This further... sets the scene for possible but to my mind artificial conflicts of interest between mother and baby in pregnancy, birth and parenting."[8]

Additional authors:

Beverly Lawrence Beech[1]

David Blake and Rebecca Panter[6]

Nancy Evans and Michealene Risley[3]

Doris Haire[2]

Parrish Hirasaki[4]

Dr David Toms[18]

Dr Carol Phillips, DC[25]

Gloria LeMay[21]

Seth Roberts[5]

Jennifer Margulis, PhD[45]

Kelly Brogan, MD[46]

Please read these authors, and others. They provide clarity, insights, and a variety of viewpoints that make this book more understandable. They can be found online and via my references. I will try not to repeat them.

I begin with a historical summary of DUS machine intensities.

FDA Intensity Limit, 1991

Much criticism has focused on the Food and Drug Administration (FDA), its regulatory changes during 1991 when it raised the allowable intensity limit for DUS machines to 720mW/cm2 SPTA. I refer to this as "FDA/1991". See the Appendix for historical verification of the year 1991.

The historical incidence of various epidemic diseases bears an obvious correlation with FDA/1991, and the symptoms and posited physiology of those diseases, such as ADHD and autism, are approximately reproducible by DUS exposure studies.

In 1991, FDA increased the regulatory limit from 94mW/cm2 to 720mW/cm2 SPTA, an increase by a factor of 8x. SPTA is an intensity parameter, the acronym for Spatial Peak Temporal Average.

The transducer contains a piezoelectric crystal that generates ultrasound.

Transducer intensity is measured in a water tank, because water is "translucent" to ultrasound, i.e., water has very little attenuation. Intensity is measured with a hydrophone (underwater microphone) as milliwatts per centimeter squared, i.e., mW/cm2 SPTA. Measurement in air would be problematic because ultrasound in the megahertz frequency range does not travel well through air.

There is an exception.

The FDA regulatory limits for intensity are "derated", i.e., they are expressed as transducer intensity estimated at the fetus or other such target, i.e., the *in situ* intensity. This is always a lesser value because attenuation is estimated with an attenuation formula in terms of intervening distance, frequency effects, biological matter, muscle, bone, and fluid.

The FDA/1991 limit of 720mW/cm2 SPTA represents much higher actual device intensity limits, as much as 3,000mW/cm2 or more, depending on the intended application, its estimated attenuated intensity being within the FDA limit.

Manufacturers use the FDA attenuation formula to estimate their devices' *in situ* intensities, to ensure they are within FDA limits during design phase and FDA approval submittal process. They rationalize and optimize device designs with maximum output intensities by use of the attenuation formula. This has resulted, since FDA/1991, in some Doppler device outputs up to 9,080mW/cm2 SPTA according to Martin (2010), though he calls that particular value a regulatory "breach".[106]

Other examples of intensity descriptions:

Whittingham (2001) estimates high intensities at the fetal target, *in situ*,

> "Spectral Doppler mode produces the highest *in situ* estimates... which exceed 5,000mW/cm2 in a third trimester minimum attenuation model, and 900mW/cm2 in a 'typical' attenuation model."[30]

According to Siddiqi and O'Brien (2001),

> "...the acoustic output from newer clinical instruments is well within the range able to produce thermal and mechanical bioeffects."[31]

Aside: "Bioeffects" means "biological effects", similar to "symptoms".

Some machines, when reviewed, have been found to be 65% above their own specified outputs. This demonstrates the weakness of the regulatory protocols.

In clinical practice, the FDA/1991 increase factor can be interpreted to be higher than 8x. Dr David Toms, radiologist, estimates higher than 1,000x, because earlier machine outputs were as low as 0.10mW/cm2. He owns a machine with 0.11mW/cm2 output, manufactured during the early 1980s. If the derating concept were applied to 0.11mW/cm2, to account for attenuation, then the increase factor could be interpreted much greater, perhaps 4,000x, as low intensity machines would be replaced in clinical practice.

Ellisman (1987) also describes a low range of machine intensities during the 1980s.

"...the published range of intensities for [common DUS] devices: 0.1 to 200 mW/cm2 SPTA..."[19]

Kimmel (1989) describes an exceedingly high upper range.

"Diagnostic ultrasound devices can have... intensities of up to 2,000mW/cm2 SPTA..."[85]

The ratio of Ellisman's "0.1" to Kimmel's 2,000mW/cm2 is 20,000x.

The ratio of Ellisman's "0.1" to the aforementioned "9,080" by Martin (2010) is 90,800x.

FDA/1991 gave the ultimate responsibility for exposure to the operators without them being sufficiently trained or regulated.

Gail ter Haar, PhD, summarizes FDA/1991.

"The change allowed intensities previously reserved only for peripheral vascular studies to be used for all studies, including first trimester scanning.

"No epidemiological or other evidence was then, or is now, available to support the *assertion of safety* at these higher exposures.

"The FDA change resulted in the widespread availability of high specification pulsed Doppler and Doppler imaging modes for uses in addition to cardiovascular applications, including obstetrics.

"Recognizing the difficulty of establishing resilient safety management for this change, the FDA decided to *pass the responsibility* for safe management to the user [operator]."[95]

The graph below summarizes an association of rising machine intensities with the incidence of autism. [Graph→]

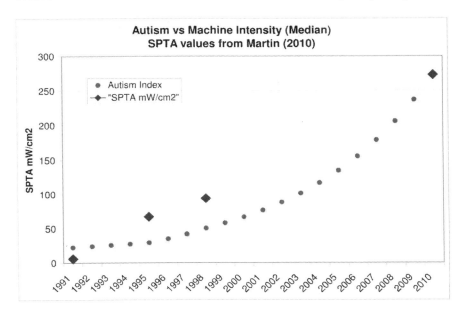

Doppler mode, mentioned above, is employed to monitor and examine blood flow properties. Can be much higher intensity than B-mode, the usual obstetric 2D gray mode. Doppler is authoritatively advertised as "harmless and painless", though well known among authorities to bring higher risk.

Nancy Evans, interviewed for the *Huffington Post*, addresses the FDA increase.

> "The FDA increased the allowable output to afford better visualization... However, the agency did not mandate appropriate training or require certification for operators of the equipment. FDA does not have the authority to regulate ultrasound facilities nor does it have adequate resources to regulate and inspect these facilities."

Before 1985, over 700 studies had described ultrasound bioeffects without any resolution of risk assessment, according to Dr Robert Bases, at Columbia University.[22]

After FDA/1991, there is an irrational disappearance of study funding in the Western realm.

The DUS industry maintains unresolved risk science. Studies that demonstrate damage are ignored, played down, and denied funding for continuation. Studies are funded with the apparent purpose of contradicting critical studies. Several ultrasound scientists have told me that their funding was denied for continuation, despite, in my view, the obvious importance of their findings. One scientist had the temerity to say that he was "disgusted" by the evaluation and funding process. Many scientists express some degree of doubt openly in their study conclusions. Caroline Rodgers has also described the lack of appropriate studies.[16]

In light of the contradictions within science and practice, critics argue that the practice of DUS should be halted until safety is assured. Professional and public ignorance continues, encultured as an excuse to maintain the practice. Industry continues on with a "Titanic Mentality", as Dr Toms has written. It admires its moonlit wake, its unblemished record, while declaring DUS harmless.

As laboratory technology has advanced tremendously, DUS studies nearly disappeared in the Western realm.

With regard to safety, Western authorities philosophically declare that, "It is impossible to prove a negative."[82]

Research Motivation

My earliest awareness of DUS hazards arrived in 1981 from Mendelsohn, and later, from articles in *Midwifery Today*. Despite the eloquence of those authors, I found it incredibly difficult to bring the topic effectively to anyone, male, female, stranger or friend, the naïveté or skeptic.

I had met a nearly insurmountable block. On a personal level I was devastated. The difficulty was nearly unfathomable. I spent much time just trying to understand the obtuse nature of my friends with regards to this topic.

A common response was an accusation of "fear mongering". Few seemed to realize that they were already thoroughly mongered by medical messages, expecting ultrasound to diminish their fear.

As far as I have been able to determine, the block is the result of ubiquitous product marketing, reaching critical mass and becoming self-supporting by the population.

Women are trained throughout their lives, directly and via imbedded advertising, to fear birth, to fear their selves, to fear complications. They are taught to see routine ultrasound as their best assurance.

Fear of birth has been part of mainstream education since ancient times. For example, Genesis 3:16, promotes the idea that human birth is an unnatural process, painful and miserable, multiplied beyond that of any other animal.

> "I will greatly multiply thy sorrow and thy conception; in sorrow thou shalt bring forth children..." (King James Version)

Some would argue that the priests of Medicine have secured this prophecy. See Dr Mendelsohn's inspired article, "The Devils Priests".

With much humor, Dr Mendelsohn reveals how fear is promoted to sell religious artifacts and rituals, though they are actually Medical products and methods, sold as fear reducers, pain eliminators, and lifesavers. The flock assumes medical protocols are backed by hard science, but their Medicine is often a political and market-driven soft science, that awes the faithful with unproven, unsafe technology, devices, radiation and pills.

The faithful take umbrage at the mere possibility that the birthing process could be more than a painful obstacle. The word, "obstetrician" insists on obstacles.

DUS, a high tech icon, is a major part of medical enculturation. It divides. It polarizes the birth process, as Sarah Buckley wrote, "ultrasound artificially splits mother from baby". This puts the medico in the middle, ready with drugs, scissors, knives, radiation, and toxic injections, tainted with conflict of interest.

George Bernard Shaw's observation rings true.

> "We have not lost our faith — we have transferred it to the medical profession."

People require authorities. Thus, I searched for authorities.

Arcana

By mid-2013, after three months research, I had found nothing definitive, i.e., virtually no human *in utero* exposure studies. I decided to look for any type of DUS study that used electrophoresis, a modern analytic technique. This is a sensitive form of chromatography, well known for its use in virus identification, the Human Genome Project, and DNA fingerprint technology. I had known of this simple technology from my prior critical research into virology. At that time, I was in a tenuous dialogue with an ultrasound scientist, from whom I requested such a study. Receiving no reply. I assumed the study likely did not exist.

My research continued nevertheless, and I soon found such a study, and it was a Chinese human study, JZhang (2002), pristine, published in English, but very low profile. It cited one other CHS, Jiao (2000), and Jiao cited other studies that lead into the tree of the entire CHS.

Truly stunned by this mass of data, puzzled by its low profile, I strove to achieve a deeper understanding of ultrasound science and politics to be able to handle this material.

Western authorities have not read the CHS. This is indicated by their oblivious comments. They are generally unaware of any human exposure studies, while declaring human studies essential to the resolution of DUS risk.[29]

4 | Human Studies Exist

The Chinese Human Studies exist. They are *in utero* human exposure studies conducted during the modern era, 1988-2011. Fetuses were exposed *in utero* to diagnostic ultrasound and the abortive matter studied in the laboratory.

So far, I have collected 48 CHS and 10 overviews that represent the involvement of approximately 100 scientists. The subjects total 2,651 women volunteering for abortions. Their abortive matter was examined with their progeny in various stages of development: 1) the ova of the female fetus, 2) the embryo, 3) the fetus. I have culled duplicate publications, though some of the overviews may be similar versions or duplicates.

With the CHS, we can say the previously unthinkable, that,

Human* in utero *exposure studies are the most abundant form of DUS research in the modern era.

The CHS are the last of their kind. Their strength, their relative purity, is derived from their relative freedom from industrial politics. They were conducted during the early bloom of modern industrial Chinese science.

They are a serendipitous byproduct of the great Chinese industrial push. A broad scientific foundation for China's industrial progress was initiated in 1984 with the establishment of the "State Key Laboratory Scheme", i.e., the institution of a variety of modern laboratories.[15]

The CHS occurred during this optimistic phase, before they could share the fate of Western critical studies, before they could be monopolized, repressed, or made devices for corporate advertising. That window of opportunity is likely now closed with China being a major manufacturer of diagnostic and therapeutic ultrasound equipment.

The fate of Western environmental science, in general, is documented by Dan Fagin and Marianne Lavelle in their book, *Toxic Deception*, published in 2002. More recently, the massive corruption of medical studies has been documented by a New York University professor of journalism, Charles Seife, in his article in *JAMA* (2013).[174].

The CHS utilized the latest scientific analytic technology, such as various biochemical analyses to reveal changes in tissue, flow cytometry to analyze and sort cell populations by their properties, and electrophoresis to visualize DNA fragmentation. Electrophoresis is a procedure where direct current is passed through a gel plate that contains samples of chemical mixtures such as DNA. The result is a graphic spread of various DNA molecular components, which are visualized and measured. Electron microscopes ("EM") were used to visualize sub-cellular damage.

The CHS surpass Western research in technical sophistication, number of subjects studied, era relevancy, subject relevancy, and volume of work.

Western critical studies, long rejected, are cited and validated by the CHS, examples being MacIntosh and Davey (1970)[28], Liebeskind (1979)[20], Saad and Williams (1982)[44], Anderson and Barrett (1979).[43]

The CHS confirm human relevance for cell studies conducted recently at Technion Institute, the prestigious research university in Haifa, Israel. Dr. Eitan Kimmel and Chen Geffen found irreversible damage at very low exposure, at a magnitude similar to Ellisman (1987), Ang (2006), and the CHS.[42]

Western authorities dominate perception of DUS throughout the world. They declare a lack of human studies as the primary reason for maintaining moot any animal or cell studies that find hazards. Western science, held in check by industrial politics, maintains stasis by means of a strong but mere sense of ongoing objective inquiry. This blocks resolution, with hundreds of animal and cell studies finding and contradicting findings of ultrasound-induced bioeffects.

As stated in the Introduction of Ellisman (1987),

> "Several reviews of the literature on ultrasound bioeffects... reveal that **most studies were inadequately designed** or inconclusive for the human medical situation; information on exposure conditions was frequently **incomplete, markedly different from diagnostic ultrasound** or in some instances sample size and follow-up were less than optimal."

The CHS resolve eight decades of Western limbo. They bring essential information — the intensity thresholds for human safety and damage. They find that low intensities and brief exposures can damage.

As low as these exposure-symptom thresholds are, as horrific their implications, I argue that the implications are worse than the Chinese scientists envision — because of the higher intensities employed by Western clinicians, and their tendency to use high intensity Doppler mode.

In the year 2000, the authority on human studies, Professor Ruo Feng[41], of the Institute of Acoustics, Nanjing University, summarized the CHS.

> "We need to reiterate that in obstetric ultrasound, diagnostic techniques should carefully adhere to a cautious scientific attitude. Specifically, abide by the following **five points:**
>
> 1) Ultrasound should **only be used for specific medical indications**.
>
> 2) Ultrasound, if used, should **strictly** adhere to the **smallest dose** principle, that is, the ultrasonic dose

should be limited to that which achieves the necessary diagnostic information under the principle of using *intensity as small* as possible, the irradiation *time as short* as possible.

3) Commercial or educational fetal ultrasound imaging should be *strictly eliminated*. Ultrasound for the *identification of fetal sex* and fetal *entertainment* imaging should be *strictly eliminated*.

4) For the best early pregnancy *[1st trimester]*, *avoid ultrasound. If unavoidable, minimize ultrasound.* Even later, during the *2nd or 3rd trimester*, limit ultrasound to *3 to 5 minutes* for sensitive areas, e.g., fetal brain, eyes, spinal cord, heart and other parts.

5) For every physician engaged in clinical ultrasound training, their training should include information on the biological effects of ultrasound and ultrasound diagnostic *dose safety knowledge*."[RFeng2000]

RFeng summarizes the same protocols slightly differently in his 1990 document: There he states that DUS should be avoided. DUS should be avoided during the 1st trimester. If specific medical conditions indicate DUS, and the hazards of DUS have been considered, then DUS should be *limited to 3 minutes or less* for sensitive organs, and limited to 5 minutes or less for other organs.[RFeng1990]

RFeng and the CHS confirm the validity of the National Institute of Health "Consensus Development Conference Statement", year 1984. That document is severely critical, declining to recommend routine DUS. Predictably, it has been pushed aside as "out of date".

Western Science: Crippled

RFeng describes the impaired state of Western science.

> "Internationally [outside of China], diagnostic ultrasound safety thresholds are studied mainly in two ways, through experimental animals and epidemiological studies. This accumulates much data, but only produces a small amount of quantitative rules, at best only serving as a reference for the diagnosis of clinical safety, but unable to provide guiding criteria.
>
> Diagnostic ultrasound safety standards should establish dosage thresholds based on a large number of human obstetric ultrasound clinical studies. That is the gap in international research, obviously a major shortcoming!"

With the CHS, he was able to place a huge exclamation mark into a scientific journal.

His assessment resembles the subtle warnings of Western authorities, for example, Dr Abramowicz's, "the lack of... human data in the field is appalling". For a while, that warning was echoed in the Wikipedia entry, "Causes of Autism", then removed.[27]

RFeng and his colleagues are the undisputed world leaders of DUS research in terms of science. It should be interesting to see how Western authorities re-engage the challenge presented by the CHS.

Global Awareness of the CHS

RFeng documents global awareness of the CHS and their unrivaled position.

> "...Yan Gong took the lead in China and completed the first clinical human study, with findings presented in

1988, in Washington DC, at the Fifth World Conference on Biomedical Ultrasound, as published. His article caused a ***positive response*** from the **international** medical community",

Gong (1988) is cited in my endnotes.[96]

The "international... positive response" is described on Dr Joseph Woo's web pages, "History of Ultrasound in China".[97]

"In 1988, Xin-Fang Wang, Yong-Chang Chou, Wang-Xue Guo, Zhi-Zhang Xu and physicist Ruo Feng were presented with the "History of Medical Ultrasound Pioneer Award" by the World Federation for Ultrasound in Medicine and Biology (WFUMB). The ceremony was held in Washington DC in the United States"

RFeng continues, describing a "special letter" of encouragement from the influential Floyd Dunn, PhD, of the United States, written April 7, 1989.

"This topic would be extremely difficult, possibly even impossible, to carry out in this country because of a prevailing view regarding abortion. If this could be carried out in your country, in my view, it would be ***a major contribution to international diagnostic ultrasound***." [emphasis added] (RFeng quotes Dunn from RFeng's earlier article, "...My Opinion", in *The Chinese Journal of Ultrasound in Medicine*, 1990, 6 (3), p210-211.)

Dunn was encouraging China's entry into DUS science with human studies, yet, as of 1989, he had not yet seen much of their results. These studies, the CHS, would eventually undermine his own work where he defends DUS. I could find no further word from Dunn or his colleagues, via the online resources of the Bioacoustics Research Laboratory or anywhere else. Here we have a complex human dilemma. Praise goes to Dunn for supporting the Chinese human studies program at its early stage.

Floyd Dunn (d. 1/24/2015) was of the highest political echelon of Western researchers, close to Nyborg, O'Brien, and Carstensen. They describe Dunn:

> "[B]iomedical ultrasound is a major industry, and basic research in the field receives a significant fraction of the NIH [National Institutes of Health] budget. No single scientist is more responsible for this success than Floyd Dunn..."[162]

In terms of industrial economics, Dunn bore a heavy responsibility.

Dunn and RFeng knew each other. Dunn was a Visiting Professor at the University of Nanjing, where RFeng was the editor of *Biomedical Ultrasound*, of Nanjing University Press.

Ostensibly, none of the Western professionals are aware of the CHS, as can be inferred from their comments listed in Chapter 7.

Dunn evidently kept quiet with regard to "a major contribution to international contribution to the development of ultrasound."

Apparently, the entire Ultrasound Community forgot about the WFUMB convention.

Ruo Feng's article (2000) was published 12 years after the WFUMB convention. Since 1990, he and his colleagues have generated many related papers. These have been limited to scientific readers in China, nevertheless, Ruo Feng put the CHS into the historical record.

The following scenario deserves consideration.

Dunn was, and his colleagues are, leaders of, "The Ultrasound Community", a term used, for example, by Thomas Nelson, in 2005, the Deputy Editor of *Journal of Ultrasound in Medicine*.[26] They are the standard bearers of DUS perception. Nelson's article, for example, is entitled, "Reporting of Bioeffects Research Results to the Ultrasound Community". It describes the scientific formalities, the difficulties of observing and interpreting DUS bioeffects.

The American Institute of Ultrasound in Medicine (AIUM) is part of WFUMB, which is under WHO. It serves as a liaison between government, industry, operators, and the public. It is able to gather, distribute and advise with regard to study funding.

Perhaps, there was an East-West cultural division?

Perhaps, the Chinese were put off by some Western etiquette?

Perhaps The Ultrasound Community was just too Western-centric.

Perhaps The Ultrasound Community felt the concerns of industry bearing upon them.

Somehow the CHS and the Western scientists did not connect.

It might be convenient to think that The Ultrasound Community overly influences the DUS dilemma, however, they are ethically concerned. They issue guidelines to reduce exposure via ALARA, and advocate for operator safety training. Unfortunately, those guidelines are often ignored, misunderstood, or viewed as an inconvenience. The FDA does not enforce guidelines, and guidelines can be difficult to implement due to the competitive business aspect of medical practice.

Dr Floyd Dunn was an Honorary Member of the Rochester Center for Biomedical Ultrasound (RCBU) at the University of Rochester Medical Center (URMC) in New York State. Other members include Dr Morton W. Miller, Emeritus Professor in the Department of Obstetrics and Gynecology at URMC, and Dr Edwin L. Carstensen, who founded and directed the RCBU. Dr Jacques S. Abramowicz is a former Director of the Ob/Gyn unit at URMC. Dr Wesley L. Nyborg (d. 2011) was a Charter Member and a Visiting Scientist at the RCBU. Industry supports these people, and their work supports industry. They may represent decades of subtle evolution under subconscious conflict of interest.

Nyborg chaired the AIUM Bioeffects Committee, which routinely issues safety threshold statements up to the present era. Figure 1 shows the 1976 and 1987 AIUM statements, where 100 mW/cm2 SPTA [spatial peak temporal average] is declared the upper safe intensity threshold. [Image→]

Excerpts from statements published by the AIUM Bioeffects Committee in 1976 and 1987.

AIUM STATEMENTS ON MAMMALIAN *IN VIVO* ULTRASONIC BIOLOGICAL EFFECTS

August 1976

In the low megahertz frequency range there have been (as of this date) no demonstrated significant biological effects in mammalian tissues exposed to intensities* below 100 mW/cm^2 ------------

*Spatial peak, temporal average as measured in a free field in water

October 1987

In the low megahertz frequency range there have been (as of this date) no independently confirmed significant biological effects in mammalian tissues exposed *in vivo* to unfocused ultrasound with intensities* below 100 mW/cm^2, or to focused^b ultrasound with intensities below 1 W/cm^2. ------

*Free field spatial peak, temporal average (SPTA) for continuous wave exposures, and for pulsed-mode exposures with pulses repeated at a frequency greater than 100 Hz.

^{b}Quarter-power (-6 dB) beam width smaller than four wavelengths or 4 mm, which ever is less at the exposure frequency.

Nyborg had misgivings about the AIUM Statements, as indicated by a brief phrase in his 2003 article:

"For lung damage in small animals at frequencies of 2 to 3 MHz, the threshold [where the] duty factor is 0.001 [is] about 33mW/cm2. This is lower than the values for the SPTA intensity cited in the 1976 and 1987 statements and therefore *indicates that the latter may be invalid* ..."[39]

Graphic Comparison

The AIUM statements are based on the results of many studies, but there are a substantial number of quality studies that contradict the AIUM statements.

In the context of several critical studies,

I graphically view the effect of the AIUM's 100mW/cm2 safety threshold intensity.

For each study, I calculate RiskThreshold values, i.e., the lower intensity found to cause damage.

I use a variation of the Exposure formula, a standard toxicology formula commonly used by ultrasound scientists.

Exposure represents the total energy radiated at the target.

Exposure = Intensity x Duration

The formula is commonsense, the greater the duration and intensity of radiation, the greater the Exposure.

Because all of these studies find a lower Exposure value that causes a type of damage, a threshold value,

I substitute the term "Exposure" with the term "RiskThreshold".

$$RiskThreshold = Intensity \times Duration$$

This formula can then be rearranged to yield Duration, given RiskThreshold and Intensity.

RiskThreshold for each study is divided by Intensity to yield Duration.

$$Duration = RiskThreshold / Intensity$$

Duration Graphs

These graphs show six durations. They show seconds of DUS exposure to cause damage given the RiskThreshold values calculated from each of six critical studies.

For the first graph, each of the six RiskThreshold values were divided by a single given intensity, AIUM's 100mW/cm2, yielding six Durations. These durations are found to be somewhat brief.

All items are placed on equal footing by comparing the *in situ* intensity values. These are the intensities measured at the target organ or fetus, or calculated to exist at that location. Ang (2006) and Ellisman (1987) measure and provide those values.

JZhang (2002), RFeng (2000), and the AIUM Statement require that the *in situ* intensities be calculated by discounting the natural attenuation of ultrasound as it travels from the transducer to the observed target (fetus, organ, etc.).[38]

Note that Ang (2006) is displayed as two studies, its 5-minute exposure, which produced positive but inconsistent results, and its 30-minute exposure, which produced positive consistent results.

In the following graph, durations are extrapolated from an intensity of 100mW/cm2 SPTA, the AIUM safety statement. [Graph→]

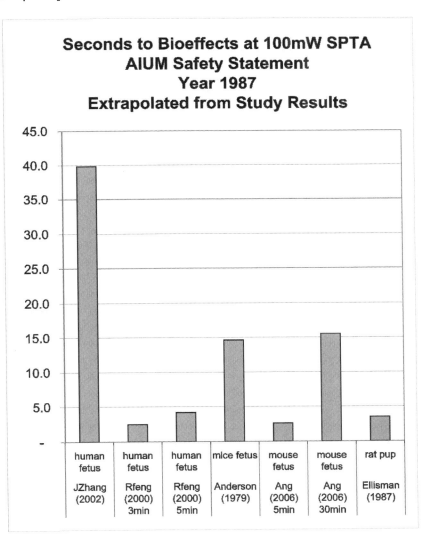

In the following graph, durations are extrapolated from an intensity of 34mW/cm2 SPTA, the average B-mode intensity in clinical practice. [Graph→]

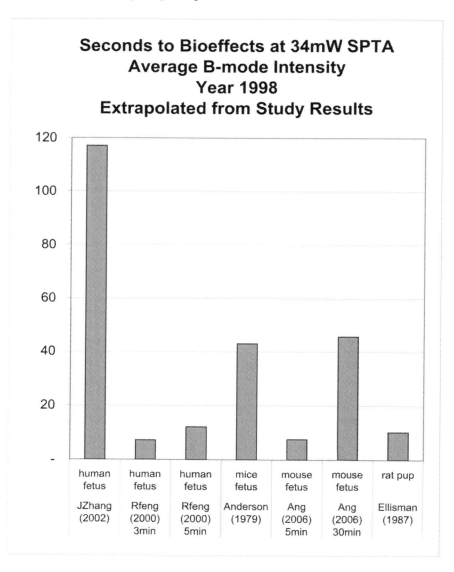

Consider these two graphs to be ballpark values, as they are extrapolations of experimental results. They are not actual experimental results. The graphs could be refined for more accuracy, for example, by accounting for dwell time (stationary transducer), however, all these studies are dwell time studies except for Ruo Feng's guidelines based on the CHS, where he warns of transabdominal sessions over 3 minutes. I doubt any further discounting would alter the message of these graphs.

The basis for these comparisons, the Exposure Formula, is from common scientific usage. It is found in the literature of Nyborg, Wiernicki, Shung, O'Brien, Siddiqi, DL Miller, Abramowicz, and others. They use the Exposure formula, or provide graphs or refer to graphs that portray Duration and Intensity relationships for damage in this simple manner. They use the formula to industrial advantage, utilizing RiskThreshold values determined from insensitive and inappropriately designed studies, as so described in the Introduction of Ellisman (1987).

There will always be margins of error, but if these graphs have any credibility, then the mainstream view must contain vast error margins.

These graphs demonstrate an extraordinary low threshold for damage causation. There may not be much room for mainstream rebuttal. The mainstream might claim Ellisman (1987) was refuted, however, I doubt they will do that, because their strategy has been to avoid mention of Ellisman. No proper refutation has ever been done, and there is no serious public discussion of Ellisman. Neither has Ang (2006) been refuted. The CHS confirm Anderson (1979, 1981) and generally confirm any critical findings.

The CHS and the critical Western animal studies are mutually confirming, all in the same ballpark. Their stated intensities, as *in situ* values, are two magnitudes away from the mainstream, which then must reside in a separate ballpark, far away.

Intensity Ratios		
5,333	FDA/1991	: Ellisman (1987)
288	AIUM/1987	: Ellisman (1987)
530	FDA/1991	: JZhang (2002)
23	AIUM/1987	: JZhang (2002)

5 | Selected Chinese Studies

In addition to RFeng (2000), there are other CHS overviews, such as ALiu (2010), and, ZJiang (2001). ZJiang provides intensity values for several of the CHS, and these are included in the following Abstracts.

If these Abstracts appear annoyingly technical, do not see that as a problem, because exposure can be simply compared to gain a sense of context, an understanding of damage thresholds.

Terms are defined for each study. Comments follow each study.

Most studies conclude with warnings about excessive duration or intensity, and that can be different from study to study due to the different parameters studied or the various methods of investigation utilized.

An Liu and Cai-Hong Li (2010)
[Topic: Overview]
[Def: Cytokines are small proteinaceous cell signaling molecules, similar in function to hormones, and important to immune and inflammatory responses.]
[Def: Apoptosis is "cell suicide", such as where unneeded cells naturally self-destruct.]

The Research Development Of Security Diagnostic Ultrasounds In Duration Of Pregnancy

Abstract: Ultrasound is biologically active and may cause the alteration and injuries in human and animal organs, tissues, cellular ultrastructures and even cytokines, ***proportional to the exposure time and intensity***. Diagnostic ultrasound results in the acute irreversible and also the reversible types of apoptosis in cells and becomes accumulated at the molecular level. In pregnancy, organs, tissues and ***cells are highly sensitive*** and subject to the environmental interference. ***Therefore***, the dosage of ***ultrasonography should be minimized*** for the pregnancy examination.

Comment

It is refreshing to read such a logical and direct statement.

Zhiyou Zhang (1994)
[Topic: Immune Dysfunction]
[Transabdominal DUS]
[Methods of observation: Microscopy]
[Intensity = 7.6mW/cm2 SPTA, 30 minutes, transducer moving, i.e., "irradiation not fixed in a range of positions."]

Study On The Effect Of Newborn Erythrocyte Immune Function Exposed To Diagnostic Ultrasonic Irradiation In Pregnant Women

Objective: The effect of newborn erythrocyte (red blood cell) immune function exposed to diagnostic ultrasonic irradiation in the pregnant women was investigated.

Results: When pregnant women during any trimester were ultrasonically irradiated once or twice, the forming rate of rosette red blood cell C3b receptors were found decreased in the newborns ($P<0.05$, $P<0.01$, $P<0.001$). The forming rate of rosette red blood cell immune complexes increased ($P<0.05$, $P<0.001$, $P<0.01$).

Conclusion: These results indicate that erythrocyte ***immune regulative systems*** of the newborns ***become dysfunctional*** after they are irradiated with ultrasound [any number of scans, any trimester].

An "Executive Summary", as a separate document, was attached to the Abstract. It details an extraordinary selection process that would be nearly impossible in the Western realm.

> The study selected the same area [locale] pregnant women, ages 24-year-old to 27 years old, 160cm tall or more. Body weight 45Kg-55Kg. Pregnant women without acute or chronic diseases.

> History: No bleeding, miscarriage, or abnormal reproductive history, no use of medicine.

> Nutritional balance: Couple in good health. No alcohol addiction, no history of exposure to hazardous occupations, solid vegetarian relatives three sides.

> No genetic diseases within generations and no abnormal reproductive history.

Comment

ZZhang supports the Western studies, Anderson and Barrett (1979), and Saad and Williams (1982), where DUS was found to be immunosuppressive.

P-values are statistical indicators that express the probability that the observed results occurred by chance.

ZZhang's P-values are very low, less than 0.001 and less than 0.01, i.e., the dose/response relation is extremely consistent.

The much higher output intensities in Western clinical practice could greatly increase the chance of a bioeffect, at the least, perhaps "Post-Ultrasound Fetal Trauma".

With ZZhang's context, DUS causation can be argued for neonatal jaundice. Previously, genetics and pharmaceuticals have been suspected for this immune system disease.

ZZhang's observation of a dysfunctional immune system could imply something worse, such as a general dysfunction of various hormonal systems, the autonomic system. Subsequent stressors to DUS exposure, such as vaccines or drugs, such as birthing drugs, could have much greater negative effects upon an infant, via DUS initiation of vulnerabilities.

Toxic synergies can be additive, or multiplicative where one stressor multiplies the effect of the prior stressor. In 1996, Qian found that ultrasound can enhance the killing effect of antibiotics "by nearly two orders of magnitude" (~100x). Microbes were killed by the combination of DUS followed by an antibiotic. Internal cell damage was determined to be the mechanism of damage, as the outer cellular structure and protective biofilm were unchanged.

The internal structure of human cell organelles bear similarities in size and function to Qian's microbes.

Vaccines contain powerful antibiotics.

DUS synergistic causation can be postulated with an example: A sonified fetus would at birth appear overtly healthy, though hormonally and intracellularly damaged. Then with subsequent application of synergistic toxins, i.e., pharmaceuticals such as muscle relaxants during birth, vaccines following birth or to the mother prenatally, or other pollutant exposure, prenatal or postnatal or early childhood, damage would rise to a more recognizable level, i.e., a more severe form of ASD, other neurological diseases, complete disablement, or death. Mild damage might not be recognizable because there are no prior characteristics to compare, no way to know the path not taken.

The view, that DUS initiates vulnerabilities, supports the heartbreaking observations of parents who describe in every detail, their children collapsing further after each succeeding vaccine dose.

A single vaccine dose may be declared technically safe by avoiding the reality of multiple synergistic stressors. The timing of vaccine and drug doses, being potentially far (weeks, months, years) from the timing of the ultrasound sessions, complicates arguments for DUS and vaccine culpability, with studies being myopic, each focused on only one toxic stressor. It appears that DUS lowers the damage threshold for subsequent toxic exposure, and with scientists myopically focused upon these subsequent exposures, DUS thereby escapes detection as a causative factor.

An example of a toxic synergy hazard: The popular flu vaccine, Flulaval, is contraindicated by the manufacturer, Glaxo, for pregnant women, nursing mothers and children, though simultaneously promoted by medicos, government, and mainstream media to everyone.[170]

Zeping Feng (2002)

[Topic: Fetus Kidney Damage]
[Transabdominal DUS]
[Methods of observation: Electron microscopy]
[Def: Ultrastructure, fine internal structure observable with electron microscopy.]
[Def: Mitochondria, organelles (within cells) that transform nutrients into cell fuel.]
[Def: Glomerulus, globular structures of entwined vessels or fibers.]
[Def: Renal, related to the kidney.]

Effects of Diagnostic Ultrasonic Wave on the Ultrastructure of the Fetal Kidney of Second Trimester of Pregnancy

Objective: To determine whether diagnostic ultrasound wave irradiation does harm to the fetus of second trimester of pregnancy and to establish the safe threshold dose.

Methods: 18 pregnant cases were randomly divided into 4 groups: I for control, and II, III, IV were irradiated on the fetal kidney before artificial abortion for 5, 10, 30 minutes respectively. All the samples were examined 48 hours later to observe the effects made on the ultrastructure of the fetal kidney.

Results: Group IV was found that irregular distribution of nuclear chromosome of the cells of the renal [kidney] glomerulus and renal tubule, the mitochondria expanded, swelled and mitochondria crest disappeared and vacuolated, the rough endoplasm reticulum expanded slightly. No changes were found in group II and III.

Conclusions: Local irradiation less than 10 min is harmless to the ultrastructure of fetal kidney.

Comment

With an electron microscope, ZFeng observed intracellular kidney damage at over 10 minutes irradiation. What would be seen as microscope technology improves?

L. Peng (2000)
[Topic: Cornea Damage]
[Transabdominal DUS]
[Methods of observation: Electron microscopy, Biochemistry]
[Machine: Hitachi EUB-40; 2.08 mW/cm2 SATA; Estimated at 6mW/cm2 SPTA]
[Def: SDH ("succinate dehydrogenase"). SDH is an enzyme complex, bound to the inner mitochondrial membrane. It is an essential component of cellular metabolism, involved in the citric acid cycle and electron transport chain.]
[Def: P-value. The probability that the observed results occurred by chance.]

Effects of Diagnostic Ultrasound Exposure To Fetal Cornea

Objective: This paper gave a preliminary study of ultrastructure and histochemistry effects of diagnostic ultrasound exposed on the fetal cornea to assess if it is harmful.

Methods: Ninety pregnant women were randomly divided into three equal groups: I (control group), II, III (irradiated for 3 and 20 minutes respectively).

Results: The continuous irradiation of diagnostic ultrasound for 3 minutes resulted in local **edema of fetal cornea** [(SDH values decreased, $P<0.05$)]: for 20 minutes resulted in the SDH values of the fetal cornea decreased ($P<0.01$). Conclusions: Diagnostic ultrasound would change the structure and function of fetal cells.

Comment

DUS changed "structure and function of fetal cells." No lower damage thresholds were investigated, i.e., a followup study should have been designed with lower exposures: 0.1 minute, 0.5 minute, 1.5 minutes, 2.0 minutes, 2.5 minutes, 3.0 minutes. The results could have been extrapolated to the higher Western intensities. That could result in exposure advice of no more than a few seconds. That could lead to regulations where only very low intensity DUS snapshots (freeze-frame) would be preferred or mandated instead of the usual stream of video images.

Given that SDH values decreased with significance of $P<0.05$ at 3 minutes, then obviously less consistent SDH decreases would occur at less than 3 minutes.

Peng's threshold values, if they were to be extrapolated to the aforementioned bar graphs, would be similar to the 30-minute exposure study version of Ang (2006).[75]

Ying-Yuan Zhu (2002)
[Topic: Neuron Damage]
[Transabdominal DUS]
[Method of observation: Electron microscopy]
[Def: B-mode is the common obstetric mode, two-dimensional images in gray.]
[Def: Lysosome is a cell organelle, membrane bound, capable of breaking down matter for disposal or digestion.]

Preliminary Study Of Effect Of Diagnostic B-Mode Ultrasound On The Ultrastructure Of Human Fetal Cerebral Neurons During Mid-Pregnancy

Objective: To study ultrastructural changes in human fetal cerebral neurons during mid-pregnancy after diagnostic B ultrasound scan.

Methods: Eight volunteer healthy women, who became pregnant for 18-25 weeks with singleton [one fetus] and asked for termination pregnancy, were randomly divided into two groups... The control group (n=4) no ultrasonography was performed. In experiment group (n=4), 30 min before labor was induced, fetal temporal cerebrum had been scanned continually for 10 min **transabdominally** by ultrasonography (3.5 MHz frequency and 70% output, SPTA= 124.1mW/cm2). All fetal cerebrum samples were prepared following routine preparation techniques for electron microscopical examination and observed under transmission electron microscope.

Results: After continuous 10 min scan, the fetal cerebral neurons had the following changes compared with the control group:

(1) Chromatins distributed irregularly, which became condensed or marginated.

(2) There were few glycogen particles in cytoplasm.

(3) Some mitochondria were swollen slightly or even vacuolated.

(4) Secondary lysosomes were observed frequently.

Conclusion: The ultrastructure of fetal cerebral neurons showed a degenerated morphology after 10 minutes scanned by diagnostic B-mode ultrasound. Since a degenerated neuron hardly regenerates, using diagnostic ultrasonography for monitoring the fetal brain, especially during the early and mid-pregnancy, should not exceed 10 minutes.

Comment

This is an important observation because the scan was the safer type, transabdominal in B-mode. Dwell time was only 10 minutes. The intensity was substantially attenuated by maternal tissue and fluid. A transvaginal examination (closer to the fetus, higher effective intensity) or Doppler mode (high intensity) would effectively bring greater hazards, possibly much greater hazards.

"Chromatins" are proteins that, essentially, maintain the nucleic acids (DNA or RNA) compact within the cell. These were damaged.

"Glycogen", in cells, serves as energy storage particles, quickly available for energy needs. Zhu found glycogen depleted, perhaps because energy was consumed by cells attempting to withstand DUS stress, or related matter was disrupted.

"Vacuolated" means, filled with vacuoles, abnormal chambers in the cell outer membranes or internal structures.

Lysosomes were "frequently observed", though these are membrane bound organelles. That is, the authors appear to be saying that lysosomes should not normally be observed so easily, that they are shaken from their membrane sites.

The phrase, "a degenerated neuron hardly regenerates", might indicate a grim humor. These scientists know they have not looked for the lower thresholds of damage below 10 minutes, yet they advise only within their observations, "should not exceed 10 minutes", apparently unable to further discuss the implications within the area below 10 minutes.

Due to the clarity of the results at 10 minutes, it can be assumed that a variety of lower damage thresholds would be found if investigated.

Typically, a Western defense would be to claim that intensity was unusually high at 124mW/cm2 SPTA. Yet, Martin (2010) lists 341mW/cm2 SPTA as the average "worst-case scenario" for machines set at B-mode.

Another typical defense is to claim that the "continual scan" is unusual, though this assumes operators follow the ALARA safety guidelines.

The opposite is well known. Western operators very often use high intensities and ignore the guidelines out of a priority concern for image quality, upon which their professional reputation depends. Their ability to adhere to guidelines is unlikely as only a minority of operators understand the safety and technical features of their machines, and generally, they do not follow the ALARA principles of minimum exposure.

Salvesen (2011) describes deplorable operator skills.

> "A questionnaire was distributed to 145 doctors, 22 sonographers and 32 midwives from nine European countries. All of them were using diagnostic ultrasound on a daily or weekly basis. The results of this study were depressing. About one third knew the meaning of MI and TI [mechanical and thermal safety indices, displayed], and only 28% knew where to find the safety indices on the screen of their own machine. More alarmingly, only 43 (22%) of 199 respondents knew how to adjust the energy output on their machine."[104]

Sheiner (2007)[37] describes dreadful operator skills, as shown in my summary table. [Table→]

"What Do Clinical Users Know Regarding Safety of Ultrasound During Pregnancy?"

CME Article, 2006, by E Sheiner, I Shoham-Vardi, JS Abramowicz

Results of a questionaire submitted to DUS operators

Obstetricians % in the polled group	81.0%
Physicians % in the polled group	63.0%
Performed routine Doppler during first trimester	18.0%
Thought low-risk pregnancy should be limited to 1 to 3 sessions	50.0%
Disapprove of keepsake/entertainment ultrasound	70.0%
Familiar with TI (thermal hazard index)	32.2%
Able to define TI properly	17.7%
Familiar with MI (mechanical hazard index)	22.0%
Know where acoustic indexes are on the display	21.0%

Among those operators who displayed competence, to what extent were they fluent? How much time would they spend deciding and finding the correct button while holding the active transducer in place?

The first trimester is an acknowledged high-risk fetal stage, yet 18% of operators admit to routine application of Doppler during the first trimester. Doppler is acknowledged to be a higher risk mode.

An AIUM warning statement, approved April 2011:

> "The use of Doppler Ultrasound during the first trimester is currently being promoted as a valuable diagnostic aid for screening... The procedure requires considerable skill, and subjects the fetus to extended periods of relatively high ultrasound exposure levels. Due to the increased risk of harm, the use of spectral Doppler ultrasound with high TI in the first trimester should be viewed with great caution."[175]

In more recent machines, intensity is shown on the machine displays, not with mW/cm2 SPTA, but with MI (Mechanical index) and TI (Thermal Index). These indexes are to assist operators in avoiding overexposure. The relationship of the indexes to SPTA is not clear. No formula can accurately convert these indexes to SPTA. Though SPTA is no longer displayed, SPTA is the most useful parameter according to Abramowicz (2011).

Doppler requires "considerable skill", including knowledge of TI and MI, yet, only 32.2% are familiar with TI, 17% were able to define TI, and only 22% were familiar with MI.

"Keepsake/entertainment ultrasound" is for family albums or theatrical entertainment where the fetus is the featured act. Medicos decry this practice, however, some medicos bond parents to their professional practice with the use of entertainment DUS, i.e., "See your cute baby." or "Look, it's a boy!"

Some medicos believe it is a medical necessity to bond the mother to her own fetus via such practice. This contributes unnecessarily to risk. The table tells us that non-medical entertainment is a well-advertised hazard within the medical community.

Machines, competing for image quality, have defaults ("presets") set very often to high intensities. Average machine worst-case scenarios, from a 2010 survey of machines, are 341mW/cm2 SPTA for B-mode, the common obstetric mode, per Martin(2010).[ref106] The range of worst-case values was 19.8mW/cm2 to 1,100 mW/cm2. Meanwhile, some experts, while claiming DUS absolutely harmless, declare less than 10mW/cm2 for B-mode.[176]

Though FDA limits DUS to a derated 720mW/cm2 SPTA, actual exposure depends on the operator's judgment. Some Western experts actually argue for high intensity limits in order to ensure marginally better imaging, and as stated, some even argue that intensity limits should be abandoned.[107]

Ying-Yuan Zhu (2005)
[Topic: Neuron Damage]
[Method of observation: Electron Microscopy of highly detailed cell inner structure]

> **Results**: As compared with the control group, the fetal cerebral temporal neuroglia cells displayed the following ultrastructural changes after 10 minutes uninterruptedly scanned in B-mode: The neuroglia cell membrane, subcellular organelles such as mitochondria, Golgi complex, and endoplasmic reticulum appeared **damaged**. Perinuclear space was **widened**. Chromatins distributed **irregularly** and markedly condensed, agglomerated, i.e., characteristic of apoptosis.

Comment

This study is similar to their preliminary study in 2002, and the results are confirmative.

Z. Feng (1996)
[Topic: Testicles, Internal Cellular Damage]
[Method of observation: Electron Microscopy]

Effects Of Diagnostic Ultrasonic Wave On The Ultrastructures of the Human Fetus Testicles

During Mid-Stage Pregnancy:

Fetuses with 20-28 weeks gestation age, destined to be aborted for whatever reasons, were divided into 4 equal groups (A, B, C, D). Before abortion, mothers of each group received different diagnostic ultrasound irradiation for 5 min., 10 min., and 30 min., accordingly, except group D, which served as an unexposed control.

Results: After abortion, microscopically, the testicles of group C showed *swollen* spermatogonia with *rarefaction* of nuclear chromosome and obscurity of mitochondria structure with reduplication of *splitting* of basal membrane, but no change was found in other groups.

Conclusion: The results indicated that radiation less than 10 minutes does no harm to the ultrastructure of fetal testicles.

Comment

Ultrasound irradiation of the testicles is recently being promoted for male contraception. That is irresponsible, because damaged sperm or testicles could propagate damaged offspring.

Zhuang Qing Song (2008)

[Topic: Chorion villi, Transvaginal DUS]
[Method of observation: Biochemical analyses]
[Def: SP, surfactant protein, resides on cell surface, binds to foreign matter.]
[Def: Villi, the capillary-containing hair-like structures from the chorion surface that interface with the maternal structure after implantation and subsequent development of the embryonic circulatory system. The villi ensure maximum fluidic exchange between maternal and fetal blood. The villi are essential to the fetus in the early stages, and gone by the 16-20 gestational weeks.]

Vaginal Ultrasound in Early Pregnancy on Embryo Villi Apoptosis

Objective: To investigate the ***transvaginal*** ultrasound irradiation time on the villi in human early embryonic cell apoptosis in order to limit the clinical vaginal ultrasound to provide new evidence.

Methods: Abortion scheduled for 60 healthy women in early pregnancy divided into control group (without irradiation), radiation 3, 5, 10 min group, application of the probe frequency of 5.0 MHz vaginal ultrasound, gestational sac at different times of continuous irradiation. 24 h after irradiation induced abortion to take down [the fetal matter].

[Biochemical tests are listed:] By terminal deoxynucleotidyl transferase-mediated *in situ* end labeling (TUNEL) line of the histological detection of apoptosis, immunohistochemistry (SP) testing and promote / anti-apoptotic gene Bax and Bcl 2 protein in tissue.

Results: In the control group a small amount of chorionic villi cells apoptosis exist, ***irradiation increased the number*** of apoptotic cells; irradiation 3 min group showed an increase in the number of apoptotic cells, compared with the control group.

Comment: Within the study's body text, the language is more severe:

From the point of view of apoptosis, vaginal ultrasound early pregnancy embryo of the time within 3 min is absolutely safe. As the irradiation duration increased, villi cell apoptosis increased, that is, the effect is time-dependent for homologous villi and embryonic tissue. To some extent, the damage to the villi reflects damage to the embryos.

Therefore, during clinical sessions upon the gestational region in early human pregnancy, transvaginal ultrasound should be cautious. Avoid dwell time [the stationary transducer]. Keep ultrasound duration as much as possible within 3 min.

Q. L. Qu (2008)
[Topic: Chorion villi, Transvaginal DUS]
[Method of observation: Biochemical analyses]
[Def: A transducer is a piezoelectric crystal that oscillates at megahertz frequency, i.e., the DUS transmitter, the probe.]
[Def: TVU is transvaginal ultrasound.]

The Effect Of Transvaginal Ultrasonography On The Apoptosis Of Chorionic Villi In The First-Trimester Pregnancy

Objective: To investigate the effect of *transvaginal* U/S on the apoptosis of chorionic villi cells in first-trimester pregnancy.

Methods: 60 healthy women in first-trimester pregnancy were randomly divided into 4 groups according to different exposure time: control group, 3min, 5 min and

10 min. Gestation sacs were irradiated by TVU with 5.0-MHz transducer. The chorionic villi were collected 24 hours after exposure. The apoptosis of chorionic villi cells were analyzed by TUNEL. The expression of Bax and Bcl-2 proteins were analyzed by immuno-histo-chemistry.

Results: The number of apoptosis cells of the chorionic villi were increased according to the time of exposure. In contrast with the control group and 3 min groups, the apoptosis cells were ***increased significantly*** in 5 min and 10 min groups ($P < 0.01$). There was no difference between control group and 3 min group ($P > 0.05$). The expression of Bax protein in syncytiotrophoblasts and cytotrophoblasts were increased significantly in 10 min group ($P < 0.01$). The expression of Bc-2 decreased in 3 min, 5 min and 10 min groups in contrast with control group, but there were no difference between the four groups ($P > 0.05$).

Conclusions: In the early pregnancy stage, it is safe to expose the fetus to TVU within 3 minutes. And ***it is almost safe*** within 5 minutes. But the exposure to TVU should not be longer than 10 minutes.

Comment

These scientists conclude that transvaginal DUS is safe for the fetus at less than 3 minutes, not safe over 5 minutes, and absolutely not safe over 10 minutes.

Qu's results are strong evidence of DUS hazards, however they might have been stronger if they did not dismiss results in the 3-minute group by requiring a strict cutoff of discussion as determined by a P-value greater than 0.05, i.e., $P > 0.05$. Low P-values indicate "statistical significance". By convention, environmental causation studies that produce results with $P > 0.05$ are often dismissed as "insignificant".

P-values, such as the famous "0.05", represent the probability that the observed results occurred by chance. P-values relate to the consistency of the observed results in terms of the hypothesis. Inconsistent results are given less weight. Data weighting is important but as a strict cut-off without discussion, it is an intellectual hazard.

Qu dismisses results where their P-value is over 0.05. Dismissing results, based on a strict P-value cutoff, is not ethical according to many statisticians. For instance, what are the results where P=0.06? That is almost the same as the acceptable P=0.05. What are the patterns of the observed results, their relation to increasing P-values, their relation to the gravity of the topic?

Parallel: If a study predicted the End-Of-The-World by next week, with a P-value of 0.09, there would be many very concerned people, including DUS scientists and operators. To a parent, the issue of an autistic child is similarly important.

Schmidt & Hunter (2002), on statistical significance:

> Significance testing almost invariably retards the search for knowledge by producing false conclusions about research literature... [and such tests] are a disastrous method for testing hypotheses.[72]

Andrew Gelman and Hal Stern, in "The Difference Between Significant and Not Significant is not Itself Statistically Significant" (2006):

> By now, nearly all introductory texts point out that statistical significance does not equal practical importance.

Qu's results should be taken more seriously — due to the low enough P-values, the clarity of the pattern, and the vital importance of the DUS causation hypothesis under the Cautionary Principle, "Better safe than sorry."

Professionals commonly warn that critical studies be "viewed with caution" lest patients be "deprived of the benefits of diagnostic ultrasound", For industry's benefit, the cautionary principle is inverted.

Nevertheless, even by adhering to the strict interpretation of P-value significance, Qu found a low safety threshold of 3 minutes. In view of such certainty, we should consider that less consistent damage would likely occur at less than 3 minutes.

Commendable is the improved statistical language of McClintic (2013), the mouse study, where its behavioral tests found social patterns similar to ADHD and Autism. Observational P-values were less than 0.05, and some patterns had P-values above 0.05, which the study describes as "trending towards significance".[103]

J. Zhang (2002)
[Topic: Chorionic Villi]
[Transvaginal DUS]
[Methods of observation: Electrophoresis, biochemical analyses]

Long Dwell-Time Exposure of Human Chorionic Villi to Transvaginal Ultrasound in the First Trimester of Pregnancy Induces Activation of Caspase-3 and Cytochrome C Release

Methods: Bioeffects after exposure to ultrasound are correlated to its duration of ultrasound exposure. Although diagnostic ultrasound has been suggested to induce apoptosis, the underlying signal transduction pathway remains elusive. In this study, women in the first trimester of pregnancy were exposed to **transvaginal** diagnostic ultrasound with 5.0-MHz frequency for 0, 10, 20, or 30 minutes **[at 13mW/cm2 SPTA]**. The chorionic villi were obtained 4 hours after exposure and activation of caspase-3 and cytochrome c release were analyzed by Western blotting.

Results: Our data suggest that long-duration exposure of the first-trimester villi to transvaginal ultrasound induces activation of caspase-3 through a mitochondrial pathway, which may be a response to ***DNA or mitochondria damage***. These findings provide a molecular rationale for prudent use of ultrasound at the early stage of pregnancy. Apoptosis can be the predictor of biological effects of ultrasound. Care should be taken to minimize the duration of exposure to high-power transvaginal ultrasound.

Comment

JZhang is technically modern, meticulously conducted and written, carefully published in English, and in contemporary scientific format. It warns of "high-intensity". It utilizes low intensity (13mW/cm2).

JZhang's results satisfy strict significance testing at P<0.01 and P<0.05 for the various tests.

DUS causation for chorioamnionitis is strongly supported, despite no explicit statement by JZhang.

The study measures DNA fragmentation via electrophoresis. JZhang determines degrees of DNA fragmentation as caused at low intensity and various durations (0, 10, 20, 30 minutes). The process visualizes gross intracellular genetic damage from DUS radiation. These observations are not mentioned in the abstract or title.

The following image is my rendering and imbedded description of JZhang's electrophoresis DNA plate photo. [Image→]

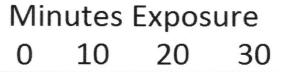

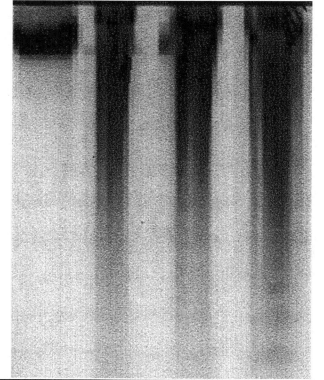

DNA Fragmentation
by obstetric ultrasound

Measured by electrophoresis

Image rendered from JZhang (2002)

"Long Dwell-Time Exposure Exposure of Human
Chorionic Villi to Transvaginal Ultrasound"
Biology of Reproduction Journal 67, 580-583 (2002)

Jim West   harvoa.org

DNA fragmentation was the result of a low 13mW/cm2 SPTA intensity applied for 10 minutes, transvaginal. Thresholds below 10 minutes were not studied.

The study discusses syncytiotrophoblast apoptosis that occurs in later gestation, thereby preempting criticism that would claim that such types of normal apoptosis are being confused with DUS-initiated apoptosis.

The strong results imply that DNA fragmentation would certainly exist below the 10-minute exposure. JZhang might be evidence for the No Minimum Threshold. With its sensitive exploratory techniques, fragmentation might possibly be detected in the area of one minute or less, putting JZhang in the Ellisman (1987) exposure ballpark.

The long-term emerging epidemics of childhood cancer seems evident via JZhang. It is generally believed that the primary cause of cancer is DNA damage. DUS should be considered as the obvious relevant causative stressor, directly or as a synergist.

JZhang is not discussed publicly, despite similar modern Western studies receiving minimal discussion, such as Stanton (2001)[77], and Ang (2006). JZhang could open up the floodgates to the Chinese human studies. I have been informed that, as a result of my lobbying efforts, JZhang is now being discussed and will definitely be reviewed in a science journal, details forthcoming.

T. Jiao (2000)
[Topic: Chorion villi]
[Transvaginal vs Abdominal DUS]
[Methods of observation: Biochemical analyses, electron microscopy, and SCE analysis.]
[Def: SCE (Sister Chromatid Exchange) analysis detects genetic damage.]
[Def: SOD (superoxide dismutase) is an antioxidant, reduces

free radicals.]

[Def: MDA (malondialdehyde) is a product of fat, lipid, oxidization.]

Influence of Sonographic Examination On Embryo Villi During Early Pregnancy

Objective: To evaluate the effects of sonographic examination on embryo villi during early pregnancy.

Methods: Eighty early pregnant women intended for artificial abortion were divided into 4 groups: Group I served as control, the remaining 3 groups underwent pelvic sonographic examination ***transabdominally*** for 10 minutes (Group II), ***transvaginally*** for 3 minutes (Group III) or for 10 minutes (Group IV) respectively.

After 1 hour embryo villi were obtained through artificial abortion and examined by electron microscopy, biochemical methods and sister chromatid exchanges (SCE).

Results: In Group IV, but not Group II, III, the embryo microvilli were found broken, lost and disarranged. The rough endoplasmic reticulum of trophoblasts expanded. Their malondialdehyde levels increased while the superoxide dismutase (SOD) decreased as compared with control (P<0.01).

There was no difference of SCE among these 4 groups.

Conclusions: It is recommended that sonographic examination should be done through abdominal approach for shorter than 10 minutes during early stage of pregnancy.

Comment

Both abdominal and vaginal DUS were studied by biochemical tests and electron microscopy, studied for their ability to damage the chorion villi. The Conclusion warns of abdominal DUS above 10 minutes, and politely does not even mention transvaginal DUS.

Gao (1996)

[Topic: Chorion villi, B-Mode and Color Doppler]
[Transabdominal DUS]
[Method of observation: Electron microscopy]
[ZJiang: B-mode, range of intensities tested: 0 to 7mW/cm2 SPTA, 30 minutes.
[Exposure required to produce obvious effects: 1.8mW/cm2 SPTA, 30 minutes.]
[Def: Vacuoles are chambers in cell walls or tissue, a form of damage.]

Effect Of Diagnostic B-Mode Ultrasound On The Embryo Villi Tissues

Objective: To evaluate the effects of diagnostic ultrasound on villus ultrastructure of early pregnancy.

Results: Expansion of perinuclear space in cytotrophoblasts and syncytiotrophoblasts, enlargement of rough endoplasmic reticulum, and vacuolization in the cytoplasm were found in Group II [B-mode] and III [Color Doppler].

Conclusions: The present study showed that the main **injured sites** after exposure to ultrasound were the plasma membrane and suborganelles. These changes were not observed within 3 days.

Comment

Cell internal structures are injured, according to visual inspection.

The low intensity of 0.7mW/cm2 as SPTA, for 30 minutes, puts Gao just below Ruo Feng's "Safe" threshold, when compared in terms of the Exposure formula.

Xiuli Han (1995)
[Topic: Chorionic villi, B-Mode]
[Transabdominal DUS]
[Method: Electron microscopy]
[Machine: Hitachi Aloka SSD-620, output intensity not found. The Aloka was first marketed in 1988, before FDA/1991, thus estimated to be no more than the intensity of Gao (1996), i.e., 0.7mW/cm2 SPTA.]
[Def: Necrotic, like death, dying, due to trauma or damage.]
[Def: Epithelium cells protect, adsorb, secrete.]

Effect of Diagnostic B-Mode On Embryo Villi Tissues

Under various durations of ultrasonic examination the ultrastructure of the villi tissues of 40 maternal cases with embryo were studied.

Results: We have found that the longer the exposure time in B-mode ultrasound examinations, the more obvious the villi tissues change. The change of group A within 5 minutes radiation was not obvious. The villi epithelium cells of group B, C and D for 10, 20 and 30 minutes radiation were swelling, *degenerating* and *necrotic*.

Conclusion: So we should inform that women who continue pregnancy should be full of their bladders at the time of ultrasonic examination, and examinations should be short exposure, avoiding repeated radiation. B-mode ultrasound examination for less than 5 minutes appeared to be safe. The stationary transducer on a fixed area **should be limited** to less than 1 minute.

Comment

The word "bladders" refers to "urine bladders" which when full, increase the distance between fetus and transducer. The CHS often advise women to have a full bladder before submitting to DUS.

Advice: The transducer should not dwell on an area for more than one minute. Dwell, "fixed area", and stationary transducer relate to each other.

Examinations should be brief. Avoid multiple examinations.

At 5 minutes exposure with a moving transducer, approximating the clinical scenario, the villi of Group A "changed" but the changes were "not obvious". That's like a Western study saying that bioeffects were observed but that the observations are not statistically significant, $P>0.05$.

G. N. Huang (1994)
[Topic: Chorionic villi, 1st Trimester]
[Transabdominal DUS]
[Method: Biochemical tests and electron microscope.]
[Def: SOD is superoxide dismutase, a protective antioxidant.]
[Def: MDA is a sign of oxidative stress, a byproduct of oxidation of lipids, fats.]
[Def: Mitochondrion are cell organelles that synthesize fuel for the cell.]

Biological Effects Of Diagnostic Ultrasound On Embryo in First Trimester of Pregnancy

Biological effects of diagnostic ultrasound on the embryo during first trimester of pregnancy were studied. Normal pregnant women who had asked for induced abortion with gestational age of 6-8 weeks were recruited.

Embryos *in utero* were exposed to the diagnostic ultrasound for 5, 10 and 30 minutes respectively. Surgical evacuations were performed 5, 15, 24 and 48 hours after exposure and chorionic villi were obtained. The villi were determined for 4 lysosomal enzymes, malondialdehyde (MDA), and superoxide dismutase (SOD); and sister chromatid exchange [SCE] and the ultrastructure of the villi were studied as well.

Results: In comparison to the normal non-exposure group, the results showed various degrees of changes in lysosomal enzymes, MDA, SOD and ultrastructure of the villi in those exposed to ultrasound 10 and 30 minutes, and most significant changes were observed in the latter group. These included the hyper-reaction of lipid peroxides; increased activities of some lysosomal enzymes; reduced SOD activity; and vesiculation and ***aberration*** of some mitochondrion, and also ***transformation*** or ***disappearance*** of some microvilli in the ultrastructure.

Comment

Huang found, via biochemistry and electron microscopy, "various degrees of changes... [after exposing 1st-trimester fetuses to for durations ranging from] 5, 10 and 30 minutes".

Sha (1992)

[Topic: Chorionic villi]
[Transabdominal DUS]
[Method of observation: Electron microscope.]
[Def: Pyknosis is condensation and reduction in the size of a cell or cell nucleus, the terminus of necrosis or apoptosis.]

Effect of Diagnostic Ultrasonic Waves on Embryonic Ultrastructure in Early Pregnancy

Changes in ultrastructure of human uterine villi exposed to diagnostic ultrasonic waves were investigated. Fifteen healthy pregnant women with gestational ages of 6 to 8 weeks were divided into three groups: Group A (the unexposed control), Group B and Group C, and continuously exposed to diagnostic ultrasound for 10 and 30 minutes respectively for Groups B and C.

Results: Pyknosis, ***disintegration***, and increased vacuolization of the syntrophoblast cells; ***necrosis*** in part of the villi; found in Group C. Only slight such changes were found in Group B.

6 | Apoptosis vs Necrosis

By convention, studies often contain the word "apoptosis", which means "programmed cell suicide". It refers to the natural death of cells. A parallel would be: Leaves *falling in autumn*.

"Necrosis" is the traditional word that simply means cellular death due to damage from a stressor. A parallel would be: Leaves *falling in spring or summer* as the result of damage by toxic stressors. Examples of stressors are powerline EMF, ultrasound, air pollution, vaccines, and pharmaceuticals.

"Apoptosis" is a valid word, but it can be Orwellian, used as an indirect, inwardly pointing term, providing a semantic escape route away from the topic of industrial toxic causation. Similarly, terms such as "allergy", "chemical sensitivity", and "drug abuse", keep culpability focused upon the poisoned victim, his genes, his behavior.

This can be illustrated with absurd extremes. One could say, "She is allergic or hypersensitive to arsenic." "Allergy" protects industry. Without this semantic option, diagnosticians could more easily indict chronic poisoning or multi-source poisoning. The word contributes to the protective umbrella of industrial propaganda, where determination of cause is claimed to be difficult, a mystery. Allergies can be more than innate sensitivities. These might more likely be symptoms of poisoning, hormonal responses to poisoning.

Such terms inevitably lead to genetic rather than environmental discussions. Industry won't object to that. The use of the direct words, "necrosis" and "damage", could diminish the chances of having a paper accepted.

A Mild Critique

I argue here that in the 5 of the 15 selected studies listed in Chapter 5, the word "apoptosis" is used only because of the necessity of science politics, i.e., to get published.

Nevertheless,

The word "apoptosis", though misleading, does not substantially diminish the importance of the study results.

I continue this argument against apoptosis, to maintain intellectual cleanliness, to maintain the potential for intellectual progress in this arena.

By choosing "apoptosis", a study places the possibility of personal weakness at center stage. It puts industry, as much as possible, offstage, protecting industry and enabling the potential for sales of medical products.

The word "apoptosis" is useful for pharma, because with it, pharma can declare the development of products to prevent apoptosis, interpreting apoptosis as the result of a personal deficiency, as a genetic problem. This explains the dominance of "genetics" as the most funded research paradigm for autism causation.

The 15 studies describe damage, injury, harm or dysfunction, with observations of system dysfunction or cellular disappearance, disintegration, pyknosis, vacuolization, splitting, and swelling.

One study describes immune system "dysfunction".

Five studies describe cellular damage as a form of "apoptosis".

Two studies describe cellular damage as a form of "necrosis".

Seven studies describe cellular damage without categorizing as "apoptosis" or "necrosis".

It is a credit to Chinese science, that nine studies do not use "apoptosis".

The Five Studies

Here is a critique of the five studies that use the word "apoptosis".

An Liu and Cai-Hong Li (2010)

This is a fine overview, though it also stays with the politically correct word, "apoptosis" (natural death), as opposed to what, in my view, is actually happening, "necrosis" (death from damage).

Ying-Yuan Zhu (2005)

This study of neuron damage uses the phrase "changes characteristic of apoptosis".

Zhuang Qing Song (2008)

This is a study of chorionic villi during early pregnancy, and it categorizes observed damage as "apoptotic cells".

Q. L. Qu (2008)

This is a study of chorionic villi during the first trimester, and it categorizes observations as "apoptosis cells".

J. Zhang (2002)

This is a detailed study of embryo chorionic villi, describing biochemical responses and DNA fragmentation, the result of ultrasound exposure that could "induce apoptosis".

I expand my critique of the word "apoptosis" here, because JZhang's observations are so abundant, clear and detailed.

JZhang uses the word "apoptosis" in accordance to the safe political trend, despite having insufficient evidence to prove the complex idea of "apoptosis" (triggered natural death) over the simple idea of "necrosis" (death from damage).

Refer to Roche (2004) and Rock(2008) to compare the properties of necrosis vs apoptosis.[178]

With those properties, we can discern that JZhang's electrophoresis plate proves he is actually finding necrosis and not apoptosis. He found destruction, a randomized structure, a DNA smear, which is typical of necrotic damage. Apoptosis would have maintained the typical DNA helix "ladder" structural pattern, and that would be evident in the electrophoresis plate image.

Choosing apoptosis over necrosis is difficult because both can occur at the same time. It is also difficult because apoptosis is the much more complex paradigm. Why would apoptosis be such a popular choice if it were not for intellectual politics?

Necrosis actually best describes JZhang, in light of Roche (2004):

> "Necrosis begins with an impairment of the cell's ability to maintain homeostasis, leading to an influx of water and extracellular ions. Intracellular organelles, most notably the mitochondria, and the entire cell swell and rupture (cell lysis)."

Necrosis is the obvious scenario, per Rock (2008):

> "...necrotic cell death arises from potentially dangerous situations to the host, while apoptotic death does not."[177]

Pay Dirt

Here's the intellectual profit, the payoff from using the proper word. We can now see a clearer and simpler paradigm for chorioamnionitis causation:

Chorioamnionitis, an *inflammation* of the chorioamnion region, is the result of DUS-induced necrosis, because, as Rock (2008) informs us,

> "...*necrotic cell death* is often associated with... an intense *inflammatory* response."

7 | Western Authorities "No Human Studies"

Catch-22 A and B

Western authorities declare DUS harmless via two Catch-22s:

A) Few Modern Studies Exist

1) Few modern studies exist of any type.

2) Older studies are imperfect and/or contradicted.

3) Analytic techniques are outdated.

4) Without modern studies, risk cannot be confirmed.

B) No Human Studies

1) Ethics preclude human studies, *in utero*.

2 Human studies, *in utero*, do not exist (with a few weak exceptions).

3) Without human studies, risk cannot be confirmed.

Examples

J. S. Abramowicz, MD (2012)[131]

> "Have there been descriptions of harmful effects of DUS in humans who were insonated *in utero*? The answer appears to be no..."

Abramowicz "appears" to be unaware of human studies. Perhaps he means, "appears to the public", yet, online forums contain heart-wrenching descriptions of damaged children by exceedingly attentive mothers who recount careless and excessive DUS, as exemplified within the forum topics found at website, *The Thinking Mom's Revolution*.[127]

H. Shankar, PhD and Pagel, MD, PhD (2011)[81]

"The potential *for ultrasound to cause adverse effects in experimental animals is well established*, but whether similar effects also occur with humans in susceptible tissue (e.g., neural) requires further investigation... [N]o human investigations conducted to date have documented major physiologic consequences of ultrasound exposed during imaging... The relative safety of ultrasound has been well established based on its use... over several decades... One could *postulate* that *humans are resistant* to ultrasound-related biologic effects..."

Why "postulate" when the CHS *empirically* demonstrate that humans are vulnerable to ultrasound-related biologic effects?

EFSUMB (quoted by Gail ter Haar, PhD, 2011)[ref82]

"Biological effects of non-thermal origin have been reported in animals but, to date, no such effects have been demonstrated in humans..."

Gail ter Haar, a DUS safety expert, appears oblivious to the CHS and even to the Western human studies described earlier, in 2002, by the FDA's Marinac (see below).

M. E. Stratmeyer, PhD (2008), FDA[83] with Greenleaf, Dalecki, and Salvesen

"To date, bioeffects studies in humans do not substantiate a causal relationship between diagnostic ultrasound exposure during pregnancy and adverse biological effects to the fetus."

How can Stratmeyer not know that modern human studies usually find DUS bioeffects? Like the others, he doesn't reference human studies. He appears oblivious to the CHS.

Douglas L. Miller, PhD (2008)[84]

DLMiller's article is titled, "Safety Assurance in Obstetrical Ultrasound". This is an excellent and highly informative article. It requires, though, a close reading.

> "There has been little or **no subsequent research** [since 1992] with the modern obstetrical ultrasound machines... The assurance of safety for obstetrical ultrasound therefore is supported by three ongoing means: (i) review of a substantial but uncoordinated bioeffect research literature, (ii) the theoretical evaluation of diagnostic ultrasound exposure in terms of thermal and nonthermal mechanisms for bioeffects, and (iii) the **skill and knowledge** of professional sonographers. At this time, there is **no specific reason** to suspect that there is any significant health risk to the fetus..."

DLMiller is presenting the problematic history of ultrasound safety as if it isn't a problem.

In so doing, he ignores Western animal studies, Stanton (2001) and Ang (2006) and Ellisman (1987), and he ignores the CHS (1988-2011). He accomplishes this with the phrase, "[N]o subsequent research with the modern... machines..." Even if the CHS did not exist, he still gives the impression that modern studies are required, with "no subsequent research", bypassing the important earlier studies conducted before FDA/1991, even though many of those were conducted at low intensities, which would make them relevant to any subsequent era of higher intensities.

He ignores a common DUS hazard, operator ignorance, with, "[T]he skill and knowledge of professional sonographers..."

He seems obtuse, with "[T]here is no specific reason to suspect... any significant health risk to the fetus..."

His paragraph can be viewed as a semantic switch: He lists **three poor general** *reasons* to suspect risk, as if those were positive assurances, then switches scope, declaring there is **no specific** *reason* to suspect risk.

DLMiller's article is valuable as a historical review of FDA policy, yet there are semantic problems.

To ensure clarity, I'll detail these problems.

"The assurance of safety... is supported by..."

"i)...uncoordinated bioeffect research literature..."

That is blatantly inaccurate. Research does not support an assurance of safety. The word "uncoordinated" is a semantic escape hatch.

"ii)...theoretical evaluation..."

"Theoretical evaluations" cannot assure safety — with funding canceled for critical experiments and discussion avoided. Theories require data.

"iii) The skill and knowledge of professional sonographers..."

How can that be anything but misrepresentation or improper sarcasm? He surely knows that sonographers tend to be deficient in safety skills and concerns. What is a "professional sonographer"? How is a patient, the ultimate consumer, or anyone else, supposed to recognize a "skilled and knowledgeable sonographer"?

He concedes elsewhere in his article,

> "[S]afety information can be scattered, confusing, or subject to commercial conflicts of interest."

As he continues, he resolves those timeless problems in industry's favor. See the original document for detail.

He argues against ALARA while mischaracterizing sonographer judgment and skill. ALARA is the acronym for the low exposure guideline, "As Low As Reasonably Allowable".

> "Prudent use implies that medically indicated diagnostic ultrasound examination in obstetrics should not be withheld or modified from the optimum imaging protocols based on safety considerations... Through the judgment and skill of professional sonographers, the prudent use principle provides further overall assurance of safety in obstetrical ultrasound."

He puts image quality before ultrasound safety, reminding us that safety is assured by the vague and unregulated "use principle". His article is nevertheless skillful and valuable as it does tell us the historical truth through a maze of safe language. It's available online, a worthy read.

J. S. Abramowicz, MD (2007)[86]

> "There is very little data on fetal exposure in the human during diagnostic ultrasound, but the lack of... human data in the field is appalling... as is the lack of knowledge of the end users."

Abramowicz is a DUS expert and a DUS promoter, featured in advertisements by Philips and Siemens. He often appears to safeguard himself by reminding us of the hazardous realities, though never going beyond a blush and a swoon. Nevertheless, he should be thanked. His material is relatively bold, revealing and informative.

While the word, "appalling" is a dramatic concession, it also serves to hide the prevalence of human data, the CHS.

W. O'Brien, PhD (2004)[88]

> "People have been studying the effect of ultrasound on development since the 1970s... We've not seen anything when levels equivalent to those allowed for humans are used." [As quoted by Jim Giles in *Nature Journal*.]

O'Brien appears unaware of the principal body of modern ultrasound science, the human *in utero* studies.

NCRP: S. Miller, with Ziskin PhD, Nyborg PhD (2003)[89]

> "Part of the challenge in determining the effects of ultrasound is that researchers ***cannot, ethically, conduct*** laboratory experiments on human beings."

Supreme ethical concern for humans serves to avoid important discussion of human studies.

Certainly, discussing human studies is ethical. Avoiding them is unethical.

Ethical is the study of human abortive matter. Abortions are already ubiquitous, routine, voluntary, ethical, politically correct, and legal. There would be no need to schedule women for abortions for a specific study, because human birth matter is routinely disposed. Birth matter should merely be rerouted from the trash to the pathology laboratory and with a priority for toxicology, i.e., required would be a review of records, X-rays, DUS, vaccines, antibiotics, etc.

Records should be required for any pharmaceutical or irradiative procedure performed upon a pregnant woman. Would this slow down medical work or make it more costly? Software already can record sessions, including DVD image recordings, for each patient. An accurate awareness of DUS risk should lower human damage and related cost. For example, if a child is born with eye disease, DUS sessions could be reviewed for excessive dwell time and intensity.

A busy industry of chorio, amnio, and placental pathology already thrives, with books, journals, and dedicated diagnosticians. It should include DUS toxicology in its pathology, but that would threaten the practice of DUS and pathology, and the vast array of related business.

D. Marinac-Dabic (FDA) (2002)[90]

> "Two studies on women immediately before an elective abortion have demonstrated morphologic changes in the plasma membrane and suborganelles under high doses of ultrasound exposure. Such approaches are not viewed as ethical in many countries."

Marinac's "two studies on women" are Huang (1994), and, Cardinale (1991).

Dangerous semantic games seem apparent.

The two studies are rarely discussed, and Marinac avoids discussion too, by dismissing them with a pretense to high ethics, and by claiming "high doses".

Marinac conjures horrific scenes of "studies on women immediately before an elective abortion...", yet no such thing was done.

These studies are ethically safe, as they studied abortive matter AFTER elective abortions. DUS exposure occurred before elective abortion, as is common practice before any abortion.

1) Marinac dismisses Huang (1994).

Sentence a: Marinac claims Huang uses "high doses", however, Huang used conventional transabdominal mode and found visual damage and biochemical effects at only 10 minutes exposure. The CHS generally strive to approximate clinical settings, usually with very low intensities, using clinical DUS devices. On the other hand, Western operators very often employ high intensities in the clinical settings with durations continuing far beyond 10 minutes, sometimes to 90 minutes or more, and with multiple sessions, sometimes many sessions.

Sentence b: Marinac knows that its allusion to the human study taboo "in many countries" includes Marinac's employer, the FDA. Marinac dismisses the topic studies by way of that distracting, cute, semantic sleight of hand, which hints at an admission of Marinac's relevant conflict of interest, his employer. Marinac might be trying to tell us that he "can't go there."

2) Marinac dismisses Cardinale (1991).

Sentence a: Marinac claims "high doses", though Cardinale states, "typical diagnostic exposure conditions".

Sentence b: Marinac gives a double meaning, appearing to be concerned with the ethics of,

> i) Woman victims of science.

> ii) Human DUS studies, as if, *per se*, those are hazardous.

Next, I review Cardinale (1991) to reveal that misinformative Marinac is describing misinformative Cardinale.

Cardinale (1991)
Bioeffects of Ultrasound: An Experimental Study on Human Embryos

My Comment

Cardinale (1991) is a rare Western human study.[147] It studies aborted human fetal matter with an electron microscope.

It finds DUS damage, however, it diminishes its own observations.

In general, mainstream scientists admit a self-defeating bias as a requirement, as explained by the article, "Scientific Fraud and Epidemiology", June 2013, from the website of the *International Epidemiological Association*.

> "We are of course aware of the problems of biased reporting of epidemiologic data in order to increase the chances of having the paper accepted..."[13]

Prior to Cardinale (1991), the same scientists had conducted six animal studies, finding strong evidence of DUS bioeffects.

In 1991, they recruited pregnant women who were voluntarily seeking abortions. These women were exposed to "typical diagnostic ultrasound conditions" where they were given "nominal exposure" with a transducer moving in both longitudinal and transverse directions across the abdomen, thereby reducing dwell time beyond that of a real-life DUS session by an amount not described nor discussed.

With electron microscopy, this human study finds DUS damage, yet its Conclusion diminishes those findings.

I illustrate this with…

Three Variations of the Conclusion

1) Self-Defeating Bias — Revealed in the Original Copy

"In contrast with the results of ultrasonic irradiation of the liver of the rat embryo, no effects on the liver of the human embryo were observed in this preliminary investigation. It is, of course, obvious that the irradiation conditions in the human were very different from those which were employed in the experiments on the rats. *It is reassuring* that the results of the present experiments *seem to exclude* the occurrence of untoward bioeffects involving liver tissue, despite the fact that the liver was shown to be the most sensitive structure in the animal studies. The *finding of vacuoles* within the liver cells in the human embryos was considered to be *negligible in comparison* with the extent of cytoplasmic vacuolization in the experimental animals… The complexity of the interactions, as well as incomplete understanding of the mechanisms, still makes it *impossible to come to firm conclusions about safety.* The present results, although not statistically significant, do not give any grounds for concern but *a study* of a larger number of patients with more controlled irradiation conditions would *seem to be desirable*."

Comment

Cardinale writes, "…still makes it impossible to come to firm conclusions about safety." Should not the practice of DUS be shut down until there are firm conclusions about safety?

2) Self-Contradiction — Clarified by Removing Non-Essential Text from the Conclusion

"No effects on the liver of the human embryo were observed... The finding of vacuoles within the liver cells in the human embryos was considered to be negligible."

Comment

How can "no effects" equate to "the finding of vacuoles"?

Vacuoles are dismissed by mere assertion, no discussion. It claims insignificance, but does not present the data for such a claim. Undoubtedly, some internal cell damage is occurring. The presence of vacuoles is evidence of damage, and evidence of possibly more extensive damage that would be visible with more sensitive microscopes, by scientists who were allowed to be more insightful.

The finding of vacuoles within the liver cells in the human embryos cannot be considered negligible because of the possible risk this implies to the entire world population. This human study, while not conclusive, lends support to prior critical animal studies. The important question remains — if we see vacuoles at this gross level of observation, then what other damage might be occurring within more sensitive structures? What would we find with more sensitive detection? What immeasurable trauma is occurring?

9 | Epilogue

Western authorities have demonstrated by their own statements (Chapter 7) that they are insufficiently challenged, that they are not challenging each other.

The CHS introduce a breath of fresh air.

How can anyone deny the numbers?

Simply compare the very low intensities used by the CHS, vs, the very high intensities and long durations used in Western clinical practice. Compare the low intensities used by Western critical animal studies, Ang (2006), Ellisman (1987), Anderson (1979), vs, Western clinical practice.

Simply compare CHS duration limits, RFeng's advice of 1 minute for eyes, and 3 to 5 minutes for a DUS session at low intensity, vs, unlimited Western duration limits for intensities anywhere below the relatively high intensity of 100mW/cm2, the traditional Western safety threshold.

More detailed comparisons within the clinical scenario are not given, and thus require the following, a sense of the politics and intensities within wide-ranging clinical ballpark.

Manufacturer default output intensities per machine are not published. Why withhold this essential consumer data?

Abramowicz (2011):

> "From a clinical standpoint, there is **no easy way to verify** the actual output of the instrument in use. Instruments from various manufacturers act differently. In addition, each attached transducer will generate a specific output, further complicated by which mode is being applied. When comparing modes, the SPTA [average per operator, machine] increases from B-mode

(34mW/cm2...) to M-mode to color Doppler to spectral Doppler (1,180 mW/cm2)..."[175]

He states 34 to 1,180mW/cm2 average intensity, from a reference dated 1998.

He claims "no easy way to verify actual output", but measuring and publishing such data would certainly help. Default outputs must be measured and published. The default is what the operator would most likely use. That data is unknown. Abramowicz may be referring to industrial resistance.

His statement, 34mW/cm2 average, is helpful, but only an average, not a distribution of possible intensities in use. His reference is also out of date, year 1998. Trends are ever increasing. Though Abramowicz sits on manufacturer advisory boards, even he cannot obtain default intensity values.

Martin (2010) describes several decades of rising intensity trends, finishing with,

"...manufacturers will continue to extend output levels towards the regulatory limits."

Industry pushes the limits and lobbies for limit increases. They must, as they are competing on the market. Operators are competing for the most efficient production of the best images. Would they sacrifice their reputation for safety? The machine manuals essentially state, Do Not Sacrifice Diagnostic Quality for Lower Exposure.

High intensity DUS is the industrial solution. Manufacturers avoid directly advocating high intensities in their user manuals. However, I see the power turned up to "100%" in the screen display printed example, in the Sonoline G20 Instruction Manual 2(en).pdf, page A2-12.

Additional Context

Without the default intensities, I can only indicate general intensity scenarios by quoting various statements.

Average worst-case B-mode intensities of various machine models are 341mW/cm2 SPTA, per Martin (2010). Default intensities are "very often high" according to Abramowicz. Some machine defaults have been found where the preset is at 50% of the maximum.

"Worst-case scenarios" are maximum intensities per device, which the operator can dial up.

Martin (2010) is very informative and up-to-date as of 2010, but also unable to provide default intensity values.

McClintic (2013), mentioned earlier, consistently found symptoms similar to ADHD in mice that had been exposed *in utero* to long dwell time, 30 minutes. With software behavioral monitoring, the study found DUS exposed mice moving faster than the controls in specified social situations. It describes its use of the Sonosite MicroMaxx portable machine, set to harmonic imaging mode to MI=0.8. Output was then determined to be 620mW/cm2 SPTA.

The FDA limits MI to 1.9 for fetal ultrasound. It does not require MI to even be displayed until it exceeds a value of 1.0. Thus, even knowledgeable and skilled operators could be oblivious to intensity levels until MI exceeds 1.0.

Western guidelines state that, depending on the diagnostic demands, the 720mW/cm2 SPTA.3 may be exceeded beyond the MI and TI restrictions for "limited periods of time".[23]

In general, machine manuals advise operators that they can dial up intensity levels in order to clarify images of target objects that may be obscured by intervening tissue, fluids, or distance.

The following is intensity data from two machine manuals found online. These manuals were selected out of many, for no particular reason, except for their convenient availability and detailed display of data.

Sonoline G60: System Ref Manual

The G60 machine is manufactured by Siemens. The manual describes the G60's worst-case scenarios (max SPTA) for various transducers and modes, from B-mode to Doppler. I have extracted and summarized that data.

The fetus is potentially exposed to a wide range of intensities, depending upon operator knowledge, ignorance or carelessness.

18% of operators in the poll say they routinely apply Doppler during the first trimester and a substantial percent of the operators are incompetent in various other ways.

Here are the SPTA intensities, which might be used by such operators. [Table→]

Siemens G60 System Reference Manual

Compiled by Jim West, www.harvoa.org

Max SPTA Values for
Curved and Linear Array Transducers (Probes)

Model	B-mode	M-mode	M+C	Doppler	Intended Application
CH5-2	140	220	1,300	1,300	Abdomen, Renal, Obstretric, Gyn, Periphal Vascular
C6-2	100	180	720	1,200	Abdomen, Renal, Obstretric, Gyn, Periphal Vascular
C6-3 3D	19	140	860	820	Abdomen, Renal, Obstretric, Gyn, Periphal Vascular
C8-5	150	290	780	1,400	Neonatal Cephalic, Neonatal Abdomen
5.0C50	100	250	2,800	2,700	Abdomen, Obstretric, Gyn, Pediatric
BE9-4	64	140	73	800	Endorectal, Endovagnal
EC9-4	85	170	830	1,200	Prostate, Early Obstetrics, Gynecology
EV9-4	91	220	900	1,400	Early Obstetrics, Gyn
5.0L45	170	230	1,500	1,300	Periph Vascular, Cerebrovascular, Musculoskeletal, Breast, Thyroid
7.5L70	58	250	58	1,500	Breast, Thyroid, Orthopedics, Musculoskeletal
L10-5	64	140	140	1,300	Thyroid, Breast, Testis, Cerebrovascular, Orthopedics, Musculoskeletal
VF13-5	81	170	110	1,000	Breast, Testis, Thyroid, Superficial, Musculoskeletal
VF13-5SP	81	220	110	1,000	Intraop Abdominal, Intraop Neuro, Pediatric, Small Organ, Periph Vessel, Musculoskeletal

The manual has an AIUM safety advisory document appended, however, the document is not listed in the table of contents!

GE Vivid i User Reference Manual

Extracted from Page 65:

Default Settings and Output Levels

The maximum default TI is 50% of the maximum possible TI (6.0) and the maximum default MI is 80% of the maximum possible MI (1.9).

Comment:

That apparently refers to user-settable defaults, not factory defaults, though it is not clear. The manual states that defaults are automatically set whenever a new probe, patient, or application is selected.

With manufacturers not publishing default output values, it might be wise to assume that they are equivalent to the above stated scenario. Without knowing the values, it would be risky to assume low default intensities, especially when high intensities are to the competitive advantage of the manufacturer, its sales force, customers and operators. The practice of not publishing default values brings suspicion.

Extracted from Page 194:

The following is from an AIUM safety document, advocating ALARA, appended to the manual. Emphasis is mine.

Medical Ultrasound Safety

Q. Are there other system features required by the output display standard?

A. The output display standard requires manufacturers to provide default settings on their equipment... Once the exam is underway, the user should adjust the output level as needed to ***achieve clinically adequate images*** while ***keeping the output index as low as possible***.

Q. ***Is it really that simple?*** All we need to know is the output index value?

A. ***Yes and no.*** A high index value does not always mean high risk, nor does it mean that bioeffects are actually occurring. There may be modifying factors which the index cannot take into account. But, ***high readings should always be taken seriously. Attempts should be made to reduce index values but not to the point that diagnostic quality is reduced.***

Comment

This confirms, to me at least, that image quality takes priority over exposure risk. High readings should be taken seriously, but not to the point that image quality is threatened.

A tired, busy, competitive, overburdened, ill-trained, untalented or desperate operator is less likely to sacrifice image quality for fetal safety. Higher intensities generally mean a better signal to noise ratio, leading to better image quality. Challenging sessions may be resolved with higher intensity settings. Any operator could max out all presets, to ensure optimum performance. We've all heard how hard medicos work, the long hours, the extended shifts, the difficult hospital internships, the continuum of dramatic emergencies.

Why should an operator trouble herself with the complications of safety, when she finds on page 156,

> "An excellent safety record exists in that, after decades of clinical use, there is no known instance of human injury as a result of exposure to diagnostic ultrasound."

That statement implies a statistical impossibility. With the millions of DUS session scenarios involving the risk of faulty machines, disgruntled operators, omnipresent badly trained and careless operators, it would be impossible to claim no single instance of human injury unless the reporting process is faulty. The key word is "known", meaning accepted by authorities. That authoritative statement, in exactly the same form, has been declared with regard to DDT, despite clinical descriptions of DDT poisoning in medical literature, and a massive neurological epidemic that matches the symptoms and historical presence of DDT poisoning.

Abramowicz (2012)

Abramowicz writes that intensities are very often high and operators little concerned.

> "[D]efault output power is **very often high** to allow better imaging, and end-users will, generally, keep it as such, mostly out of **lack of concern for bioeffects**. Excellent diagnostic images can be obtained at lower output powers. Until recently, the default power setting for machines from most manufacturers was high, presumably to obtain optimal images at the exam onset."

He has summarized the tragic Western position. Though his presentation is in a cool tone, the import of his message means more than words can convey. Exclamation mark.

His less technical summary:

> "In the United States, ultrasound **is not recommended** as routine in obstetrical care **by any professional organization**... [T]he vast majority of end-users (and patients) will respond that ultrasound is not X-

rays and is completely safe. In reality, there is *a*
***marked lack of knowledge*...*"*

Caveat: His peer, Gail ter Haar (2011), contradicts him, with a slight semantic shift,

> "[P]rofessional bodies convey... that there is **no reason to withhold** diagnostic ultrasound during pregnancy, provided it is performed by fully trained operators. The exception to this is the routine use of Doppler in the first trimester of pregnancy."

Recent intensity surveys: From machine to machine, transducer to transducer, pulsed Doppler ranges as high as 2,830mW/cm2, and, Color Doppler as high as 1,480mW/cm2, per Martin (2010).

Compare all of the above to Ellisman (1987) where fetal myelination was found consistently disrupted at a mere 0.135mW/cm2.

Safety requires lower intensities. Lower intensities mean somewhat lower image quality. Operators and manufacturers are competing against each other for marginally better images, and thus they are motivated to push intensities high and to push concerns about safety to the background.

Operators and manufacturers are forced into an unnecessary dog race, because, as Abramowicz notes,

> "Excellent diagnostic images can be obtained at lower output powers."

The CHS summary statements by ZJiang (2001) and RFeng (2000), "3 minutes is safe and 5 minutes is almost safe", and Xiuli Han's "less than 1 minute" for a stationary transducer, would need an adjustment to far smaller duration units, i.e., down to seconds, in view of the much higher intensities expressed above.

Toxic Synergies

Important is Qian (1996), its measurements of DUS toxic synergy. DUS should be conducted in terms of the obvious toxic synergies, e.g., vaccines, antibiotics, other pharmaceutical exposures, and industrial forms of radiation like powerline EMF, WiFi and X-rays. Otherwise, the true hazards of DUS are underestimated.

The National Vaccine Information Center,

> "CDC recommended 49 doses of 14 vaccines between day of birth and age six and 69 doses of 16 vaccines between day of birth and age 18..."[24]

Various pharmaceuticals and vaccines are advocated for pregnant and nursing women, and children, by industry and government despite warnings from the manufacturer.

Toxic synergies would multiply or add to the severity of symptoms already observed by scientists and parents.[143]

Open Debate

The reader would benefit from debate, from public discussion of the pros and cons of DUS. Currently, industrial interest dominates. It cites general mortality statistics against home birth, thereby promoting hospital routines and products.

An example of such technique is Wikipedia's argument against home birth in its "Home Birth" entry.[173]

Such statistics fail to separate the unfortunate population from the healthy aware population. They lump everyone together to produce frightening statistics, injecting fear to enforce and rationalize medical product and procedure sales.

General statistics cannot be used to rationally argue for individual birth protocols, because individual characteristics supercede general descriptions. The decision for home birth depends upon the individual character and history of parents, women and midwives. Those who have confidence and knowledge should be given positive options.

FDA/1991 Year Verification

DUS literature refers to three different years in reference to the FDA's raising of the machine intensity limit by a factor of 8x, i.e., from 94mW/cm2 to 720mW/cm2 SPTA. Some say 1992, others 1993, and here, 1991.

1991 is best because it correlates DUS more effectively with various disease epidemics.

1991 is also historical fact according to the official summary of Report 140, published by the National Council on Radiation Protection and Measurements ("NCRPM").[17]

> "In 1991, the US government relaxed their regulations and began allowing the intensity (or acoustic output) level of ultrasound used to scan the *in utero* fetus to increase almost eight times over the level that had been allowed previously. [...] Virtually all of the studies so far of *in utero* ultrasound exposure tracked babies exposed to the earlier, lower acoustic output levels, not the higher levels allowed since 1991.
>
> Thus, the NCRP concludes that, 'The comfort obtained from the absence to date of any harm based on epidemiological evidence must be tempered by the fact that there are no epidemiological studies appropriate and adequate for current clinical practice."

Note: "*in utero*... tracked babies" represents a strangely consistent trend of vagueness in this area. The phrase actually refers to retrospective population studies of DUS where some children happened to have been exposed *in utero*. The phrase does not mean rigorously designed and implemented *in utero* exposure, followed by laboratory analyses as the CHS have done. The Western mainstream apparently doesn't mind if their phraseology is misunderstood for the better.

The NCRP summary acknowledges two authorities:

> "This summary of NCRP Report No. 140 was initially prepared by Susan Katz Miller. The NCRP gratefully acknowledges her work and the technical suggestions made by Dr Marvin C. Ziskin and Dr Wesley L. Nyborg."

For decades, Nyborg was chairman of the Bioeffects Committee of the American Institute of Ultrasound in Medicine ("AIUM"), and chairman of the National Council on Radiation Protection and Measurements ("NCRPM") Scientific Committee.

AIUM is an affiliate of World Federation for Ultrasound in Medicine and Biology ("WFUMB"), which is an affiliate of World Health Organization ("WHO"). AIUM coordinates ultrasound topics between government, industry, operators, and with its regional focus, the U.S. It has a membership that includes scientists, operators, and representatives from industry and government. It provides certification, receives and advises funding, has various committees, and provides member and public information.

Bibliography
The Chinese Human Studies

Introduction

In addition to discovery and compilation of the CHS, I have extended my technical and political knowledge to be able to evaluate the data, to present and argue ultrasound causation. This process began in mid-2013 and included requests to professionals for feedback.

The CHS bibliography is presently 48 human studies and 10 overviews. There are more CHS online, but mostly of the chorioamnion region. The numerous chorioamnion studies are nevertheless very important because the status of the chorioamnion reflects the status of the fetus. DNA fragmentation within the chorioamnion would likely occur to any adjacent or interconnected biological matter.

I have not seen anything that substantially adds to the present CHS Bibliography. I anticipate there may be found through continued research, a possible total of 60 human studies and 35 animal and cell studies, looking for lower bioeffect thresholds.

One huge study is omitted from general discussion. This study employs *in utero* exposure, however, it is unique because it is not a toxicological study and it has no controls. It consists of 1,300 maternal/fetal pairs exposed to DUS, designed to demonstrate the value of DUS for detection of eye related problems. It is not able to discount DUS causation for eye damage. It serves as a promotional study for DUS. If I were to accept it, then the total human subjects would be 4,037. [Summary Table→]

Chinese Human Studies, by Category	
Chorioamnion	31
Comprehensive (Cornia, Villi)	2
Cornea Edema	1
Immune System	3
Kidney	1
Mutagenic (Cancer, Leukemia, etc)	2
Neurological	2
Ovary	2
Pituitary Gland	1
Testicles	3
Total In Utero Studies	**48**
Overviews	10
Total Human Studies	**58**

Animal Studies, Examples	15
Cell Studies, Examples	5

Chinese Human Studies, Totals	
Studies with subject counts	35
Studies without counts	13
Total in utero studies	**48**
Average subjects per study	55
Estimated missing subject count	13
Estimated TOTAL subjects	**2,651**

Possible CHS	65
Possible Total Subjects	3,590

If we include fetuses as subjects, then the number of human subjects involved in these *in utero* exposure studies would be approximately 7,200.

This bibliography will likely be reviewed by industrial and governmental representatives and boards. For certain, some elements of this work are now being professionally reviewed and taken seriously.

Nevertheless, the history of DUS guarantees that the CHS will be dismissed, diminished, or ignored by the authoritative process. Even if scientists were to embrace the CHS, industries would ignore them or use them to revolutionize product sales. The public and government, under industrial media influence, will continue as usual. The DUS market will continue to expand.

Only 5 of the 65 CHS can be found in the NIH PubMed database online. PubMed does not contain any of the CHS scientists who wrote overviews, i.e., Ruo Feng, Zong-yi Jiang, Ming Lang Peng, An Liu, or Canal Cui. Though Yan Gong brought the CHS to the world in 1988 via the WFUMB convention, his work is not listed in NIH PubMed.

PubMed does contain a tremendous number of Chinese studies promoting new medical ultrasound technology. Perhaps interested parties are assisting the PubMed librarians.

For new information and updates, join the email list at harvoa.org.

Researchers

If unable to find titles in Chinese databases, then perform internet searches with unique title fragments. A few of these studies can be found on PubMed, though crudely and without their citations. Note that some authors may be listed for multiple studies, yet with their names spelled slightly differently in different publications. Those may be translation artifacts. Text and names may be already be translated to English by software or humans.

Online translation software works fine if the science and politics is understood well enough to allow editorial cleanup.

The bibliography does not always provide URLs because sometimes these were generated by internal search engines as temporary paths, and some fixed URLs have disappeared.

Suggested online databases: CNKI, CAOD, Oriprobe, and Research Gate.

The list of Chinese study databases, at the University of Illinois: http://www.library.illinois.edu/ias/Databases/Chinese.html

The University of Illinois does not mention CNKI, a fine source for uncommon studies.

Views/Downloads

See and/or download updated bibliographies, Zotero database files (RDF), and bibliographic reports at:

http://harvoa.org/chs

Zotero is an open-source citation manager, with plug-ins for major browsers that allows citations to be handily downloaded and stored in Zotero, in a standard format from sites such as PubMed. It also has a software plug-in for MS Word that allows Zotero's formatted references to be inserted into your own work. It competes well with the best citation managers.

Once this book is published and its impact assessed, I may avail the bibliography lists at
http://harvoa.org/chs/bib

I note studies that appear as duplicates or as different published versions. I omit these from the summary numbers.

Send corrections, updates, and comments to

pub@harvoa.org

Human Studies By Category

Overviews

[CCui1998] Canal Cui, and Min Xia, "Research On The Impact Of Fetal Development B-Mode Ultrasound", *China Eugenics Journal*, April 1998. http://en.cnki.com.cn [n/a PubMed]

[RFeng1986] Ruo Feng, "The Views on the Safety of Ultrasound Imaging Diagnostic Technique in Pregnancy", Chinese Journal Of Medical Imaging Technology, February 1986. http://en.cnki.com.cn/Article_en/CJFDTOTAL-ZYXX198602004.htm. [n/a PubMed]

[RFeng1989] Ruo Feng, "Obstetric Ultrasound Image Diagnosis Latest Research Safety - To Participate In October 1988 Opinion Of The Meeting In Washington WFUMB", *Chinese Journal Of Ultrasound In Medicine*, April 1989. http://en.cnki.com.cn [n/a PubMed]

[RFeng1990] Ruo Feng, "Diagnosis Of Intrauterine Fetal Ultrasound On Embryonic Dose Safety Studies, Article: My Opinion", *Chinese Journal of Ultrasound in Medicine*, 6, no. 3 (1990): 210–11. http://en.cnki.com.cn [n/a PubMed.]

[RFeng1990b] Ruo Feng, Hua Mao Li, "Pregnancy Ultrasound Image Diagnosis Safe?", *Nature Journal*, 1990, 669–73. http://en.cnki.com.cn [n/a PubMed]

[RFeng1998] Ruo Feng, "The Safety Problem of Ultrasound Examination in Obstetrics", *Journal of CAUME*, 4, no. 2 (1998): 63–67. http://en.cnki.com.cn [n/a PubMed]

[RFeng1998b] Ruo Feng, "Biological Effects Of Ultrasound And Ultrasound Dosimetry", *Ultrasound in Medicine, Third Edition*, Beijing, Science Press, 1998, 57-74, Guo Zhou Yong, Science Editor. http://bbs.seedit.com/thread-179663-1-1.html [dead link] [n/a PubMed]

[RFeng2000] Ruo Feng, "Biological Effects Of Ultrasound And Diagnostic Ultrasound Safe Threshold Dose", Institute of Acoustics, Nanjing University, State Key Laboratory of Modern Acoustics, 2000. http://lib.cnki.net/cjfd/ZGCY200003013.html [n/a PubMed]

[RFeng2001] Zong-yi Jiang, Wu Min, "The Security Of Ultrasound Examinations For Fetus", *General Hospital Of Nanjing Military Region*, Nanjing Jiangsu 210002, China. 2001. http://en.cnki.com.cn/Article_en/CJFDTOTAL-YLSX200201010.htm [n/a PubMed]

[ALiu2010] An Liu, Cai-hong Lei, "The Research Development Of Security Diagnostic Ultrasounds In Duration Of Pregnancy", *Medical Recapitulation*. 2010 Jul. http://en.cnki.com.cn/Article_en/CJFDTOTAL-YXZS201007047.htm [n/a PubMed]

[XMa2005] Xiao-juan Ma, and Yu Wang, "Progress in Ultrasound Induced Apoptosis", Chinese Journal of Clinical Rehabilitation 15 (2005). http://en.cnki.com.cn/Article_en/CJFDTOTAL-XDKF200515069.htm [n/a PubMed]

[MPeng1997] Ming Lang Peng, Ying Kongqiu, and Ruo Feng, "Impact Of Diagnostic Ultrasound On Human Fetal Safety", *Chinese Journal of Ultrasound in Medicine,* 13, no. 8 (1997): 51–53. http://en.cnki.com.cn [n/a PubMed]

Chorioamnion

[SChen2006] Shan-shan Chen, Fei Xia, and Zi-jun Li, "Effects of Diagnostic Ultrasound on Ultrastructure of Human Villi", *Suzhou University Journal of Medical Science*, March 2006. http://en.cnki.com.cn/Article_en/CJFDTOTAL-SYXU200603035.htm [n/a PubMed] [35 women]

[YCui2001] Yunhe Cui, Xianshu Tian, and Jing Guan, "An Assessment Of The Effect Of Diagnostic Ultrasound On Human Embryos", *Journal of Jinan Medical College*, January 2001. http://en.cnki.com.cn [n/a PubMed] [120 women]

[RDong2005] Rong Di Dong, "Ultrasound Diagnosis Of Radiation Impact On The Expression Of Caspase-3,8 From Human Villus Cells", Wuhan University, 2005. http://en.cnki.com.cn [n/a PubMed] [24 women]

[LDu2000] Lian Fang Du, and Qingping Zhang, "Fas/FasL Protein Expression in First Trimester Pregnancy Trophoblast after Diagnostic Ultrasound Irradiation", *Chinese Journal Of Ultrasound In Medicine*, October 2000. http://en.cnki.com.cn [n/a PubMed] [24 women]

[LDu2001] Lianfang Du, Qingping Zhang, and Wangpeng Liu, "Apoptosis of First-Trimester Pregnancy Villi and Diagnostic Ultrasound", *Chinese Journal Of Medical Imaging Technology*, April 2001. http://en.cnki.com.cn/Article_en/CJFDTOTAL-ZYYZ200104020.htm [n/a PubMed] [24 women]

[LDu2002] Lian-fang Du, Xiaochan High, and Kan Zhou, "Human Villi Diagnostic Ultrasound Irradiation Cell P53 mRNA Bcl-2 mRNA Expression Change", *Shanxi Journal of Medicine*, May 2002. http://en.cnki.com.cn [n/a PubMed] [24 women]

[LFu2009] Lin Fu, Erdun E, Shishan Bai, and Moqi Wang, "Effect of Diagnostic Ultrasound Irradiation on Trophoblast Tnf-A and Tumor Necrosis Factor Receptor P55 Expression in First-Trimester Pregnancy", *Journal of Ultrasound in Clinical Medicine*, August 2009. http://en.cnki.com.cn/Article_en/CJFDTOTAL-LCCY200908014.htm [n/a PubMed] [60 women]

[SGao2010] Su Fang Gao and Zuo Li, "Apoptosis And Restoration Of Human Villi During First Trimester Pregnancy After Exposure To Transvaginal Ultrasound", Clinical Hospital of Tianjin Medical University, 2010. http://en.cnki.com.cn http://www.globethesis.com [n/a PubMed] [105 women]

[YGao1996] Y Gao and H Yang, "Effects Of Diagnostic Ultrasound On Villus Ultrastructure Of Early Pregnancy", *Zhong-

hua fu chan ke za zhi [Journal of Obstetrics and Gynecology], 31, no. 3 (March 1996): 156–58. http://en.cnki.com.cn http://www.ncbi.nlm.nih.gov/pubmed/8758789 [46 women]

[LHai2001] Ou Lu Hai, Li Zhang, and Dongmei, Hao, "Study On The Effect For Chorionic Villi After Ultrasonic Test By Diagnostic Dose", Chinese
Journal of Birth Health & Heredity, Shanghai Institute of Metallurgy; Materials Physics and Chemistry (Professional) PhD thesis in 2000,
January 2001. http://en.cnki.com.cn [n/a PubMed] [n/a subject count in Abstract]

[XHan1995] Xiuli Han, Hongwei Guo, and Wei Nie, "Effect Of Diagnostic B-Ultrasound On The Embryo Villi Tissues", *Chinese Journal Of Ultrasound In Medicine*, May 1995. http://en.cnki.com.cn/Article_en/CJFDTOTAL-XAYX199001032.htm [n/a PubMed] [40 women]

[ZHu2008] Zhian Hu et al., "The Effect Of Diagnostic Transvaginal Color Doppler Ultrasound On Apoptosis Of Human Chorionic Villi Cells In The First Trimester Of Pregnancy", *Journal of Ultrasound in Clinical Medicine*, October 2008. http://en.cnki.com.cn/Article_en/CJFDTOTAL-LCCY200810005.htm [n/a PubMed] [n/a subject count in Abstract].

[GHuang1994] G N Huang, C J Wang, and H Ye, "Biological Effects Of Diagnostic Ultrasound On Embryo In First Trimester Of Pregnancy", *Zhonghua fu chan ke za zhi [Journal of Obstetrics and Gynecology]*, 29, no. 7 (July 1994): 417–19, 446. http://en.cnki.com.cn http://www.ncbi.nlm.nih.gov/pubmed/?term=8001420 [n/a subject count in Abstract]

[LHuo2001] Lirong Huo, Jian tao Liang, and Yu fang Ren, "Effect of Diagnostic Ultrasound on NO and NOS in Human Intrauterine Villi in Early Pregnancy", *Journal of Shanxi Medical University*, May 2001. http://en.cnki.com.cn/Article_en/CJFDTOTAL-SXYX200105013.htm [n/a PubMed]

[LHuo2001c] Lirong Huo, Jinmin Liu, and Xianzeng Yang, "Induction of Apoptosis of Villous Cells in Early Pregnancy by Diagnostic Ultrasound", *Chinese Journal Of Ultrasound In Medicine*, December 2001. http://en.cnki.com.cn [n/a PubMed] [n/a subject count in Abstract]

[JJia1998] Jianwen Jia, Wu Zhang, and Liying Miao, "Multi-Target Evaluation of Effects on Human Early Pregnancy Villous in Uteri after Exposed to Diagnostic Ultrasound", *Chinese Journal Of Medical Imaging Technology*, January 1998. http://en.cnki.com.cn [n/a PubMed] [125 women]

[TJiao2000] Tong Jiao, L Liu, and Z Wang, "Influence of sonographic examination on embryo villi during early pregnancy", *Zhonghua fu chan ke za zhi [Journal of Obstetrics and Gynecology]*, 35, no. 7 (July 2000): 406–7. http://en.cnki.com.cn http://www.ncbi.nlm.nih.gov/pubmed/11776185 [80 women]

[WLi2002] Wei Ping Li, et al., "Effects Of Diagnostic Ultrasound On Human Villi: Ultrastructure And Hydrogen Peroxide Cytochemistry Observation", *Academic Journal of Second Military Medical University*, March 2002. http://en.cnki.com.cn [n/a PubMed] [15 women]

[ZLi2006] Zi-jun Li, Fei Xia, and Zong-ji Shen, "Detection of the Expression of Caspase-3 mRNA in Human Villi after Diagnostic Ultrasound Irradiation by RT-PCR" Reproduction & Contraception, March 2006. http://en.cnki.com.cn/Article_en/CJFDTOTAL-SZBB200603005.htm [n/a PubMed] [66 women]

[LLiu1999] Li Liu, Tong Jiao, and Zhifen Wang, "Biological Effects of Diagnostic Ultrasound on Human Embryos in Uterus", Tianjing Medical Journal, November 1999. http://en.cnki.com.cn/Article_en/CJFDTOTAL-TJYZ199911008.htm [n/a PubMed] [60 women]

[GLu1992] Guorong Lu, "Effects of Diagnostic Ultrasound on Human Embryos in Uterus", *Chinese Journal Of Ultrasound*

In Medicine, January 1992. http://www.ncbi.nlm.nih.gov/pub-med/?term=8001420 [55 women]

[JMeng1995] Jun Meng, "Effects of Vaginosonography on Human Embryonic Ultrastructure in Early Pregnancy", *Chinese Journal Of Medical Imaging Technology*, February 1995. http://en.cnki.com.cn/Article_en/CJFDTOTAL-ZYXX502.005.htm [n/a PubMed] [9 women]

[QQu2008] Qing Lan Qu and Cui Fang Hao, "The Effect Of Transvaginal Ultrasonography On The Apoptosis Of Chorionic Villi In The First-Trimester Pregnancy", Qingdao University, 2008. http://www.globethesis.com http://en.cnki.com.cn/Article_en/CJFDTOTAL-NXYX201008020.htm [n/a PubMed] [60 women]

[JQin2006] Jun-li Qin, Jian-fang Zhu, Juan-juan Xing, Zhi-an Hu, and Xiao-lin Yu, "Effect of Diagnostic Transvaginal Color Ultrasound on Apoptosis of Human Chorionic Villi Cell in the First Trimester of Pregnancy", Acta Academiae Medicinae Jiangxi, April 2006. http://en.cnki.com.cn/Article_en/CJFDTOTAL-JXYB200604036.htm [n/a PubMed] [25 women]

[ASha1992] Aiguo Sha, "Effect of Diagnostic Ultrasonic Waves on Embryonic Ultrastructure in Early Pregnancy", *Chinese Journal Of Ultrasound In Medicine,* February 1992. http://en.cnki.com.cn/Article_en/CJFDTOTAL-ZGCY199302018.htm [n/a PubMed] [15 women]

[ZQing2008] Zhuang Qing Song, Hao Ning, Hung Cuifang, Hung Wang, and Meimei Wang, "Vaginal Ultrasound Early Pregnancy on Embryo Villi Apoptosis", 2008. http://eng.hi138.com/medicine-papers/clinical-medicine-papers/201105/310704_vaginal-ultrasound-early-pregnancy-on-embryo-villi-apoptosis.asp [n/a PubMed] [60 women]

[DWang1995] Dunli Wang, "Effect of Routine Diagnostic Ultrasound on Ultrastructure of Early Pregnancy Embryonic

Villus", Chinese Journal Of Ultrasound In Medicine, December 1995. http://en.cnki.com.cn/Article_en/CJFDTOTAL-ZGCY512.020.htm. [30 women]

[YWu1986] Ye Wu and Xianting Zhou, "Study of Prenatal Diagnosis on First Trimester of Pregnancy Six Enzymes Determination for Chorionic Villi Samples", *Acta Genetica Sinica*, February 1986. http://en.cnki.com.cn [n/a PubMed] [187 women]

[FXia2006] Fei Xia, Zhi-jun Li, Jun He, and Zong-ji Shen, "Effects of Diagnostic Transabdominal Ultrasound on Human Villi", *Journal of Chinese Physician*, September 2006. http://en.cnki.com.cn/Article_en/CJFDTOTAL-DDYS200609000.htm [n/a PubMed] [35 women]

[SLiu1995] Shu-Ying Liu, Baodong Zhang, Xiaoling Liu, Jing Ping Guo, Yuhua Rain, Was Bi Shaoping, and Zhanglan Zhi, "Effect of Diagnostic Broad Bandwidth Ultrasound on Ultrastructure of Human Intra-Uterine Villi in Early Pregnancy", *Chinese Journal of Ultrasound Imaging*, March 1995. http://en.cnki.com.cn/Article_en/CJFDTOTAL-ZHCY503.008.htm [n/a PubMed] [27 women]

[QYu2010] Qiao-Yan Yu, "The Effects Of Vagina Supersonic Radiation On The Human Early Embryo", *Ningxia Medical Journal*, October 2010. http://en.cnki.com.cn/Article_en/CJFDTOTAL-NXYX201008020.htm [n/a PubMed] [50 women]

[JZhang2002] JiaYin Zhang, et al., "Long Dwell-Time Exposure of Human Chorionic Villi to Transvaginal Ultrasound in the First Trimester of Pregnancy Induces Activation of Caspase-3 and Cytochrome C Release", *Biology of Reproduction* 67, no. 2 (August 1, 2002): 580–83. http://www.biolreprod.org/content/67/2/580 ; http://www.ncbi.nlm.nih.gov/pubmed/12135899 [24 women]

[SZhang1995] Shu-Ying Zhang et al., "Ultra-wideband Diagnostic Ultrasound Influence on the Human Body and Recent

Human Villi Ultrastructure Reusable", *Chinese Journal of Ultrasound Imaging*, March 1995. http://en.cnki.com.cn [n/a PubMed] [27 women]

[CZhou2005] Chun Zhou, Dirong Dong, and Yuanzhen Zhang, "Caspase-3 and Caspase-8 Protein Expression In The First Trimester Pregnant Trophoblast After Diagnostic Ultrasound Irradiation", *Chinese Journal Of Ultrasound In Medicine*, April 2005. http://en.cnki.com.cn [n/a PubMed] [24 women]

[JZi2006] Jun Li Zi, "A Preliminary Study On The Safety Of Diagnostic Ultrasound Human Biological Effects Villi", *Suzhou University Journal of Medical Science*, 2006. http://en.cnki.com.cn [n/a PubMed] [66 women]

[ZSong2008] Zhuang Qing Song, "Vaginal Ultrasound Early Pregnancy on Embryo Villi Apoptosis", 2008. http://eng.hi138.com/medicine-papers/clinical-medicine-papers/201105/310704_vaginal-ultrasound-early-pregnancy-on-embryo-villi-apoptosis.asp [n/a PubMed] [60 women]

Comprehensive (Villi, Cornea, etc)

[LPeng1991] Lang Ming Peng, Chiu Ying Kong, Cheung Chan Sung, Yu Sun, Fung if, Tsai Wen, and Guo Nianqun, "Impact Of Diagnostic Ultrasound On Human Fetal Safety", *PLA Guangzhou Medical Junior College*, January 1991. http://en.cnki.com.cn [n/a PubMed] [90 women]

[LPeng1997] Lang Ming Peng, Qiuying Kong, and Ruo Feng, "Effects of Diagnostic Ultrasound Exposure to Human Fetus", Chinese Journal Of Ultrasound In Medicine, August 1997, http://en.cnki.com.cn/Article_en/CJFDTOTAL-ZGCY199708026.htm [n/a PubMed] [80 women]

[ZWu1998] Zhang Wu, Ying Li Miao, Guorong Lu, Shuying Wu, and Fu Shao Lin, "Multiple Indicator Ultrasound Diagnosis Of Intrauterine Pregnancy Villous Impact Assessment", *China Medical Imaging Technology*, January 1998. http://en.cnki.com.cn [n/a PubMed] [125 women]

Cornea Edema

[LPeng2000] Lang Ming Peng, Jiashong Guo, Qiuying Kong, "Effects of Diagnostic Ultrasound Exposure to Fetal Cornea". *Journal of Branch Campus of the First Military Medical.* 2000 Feb. http://en.cnki.com.cn/Article_en/CJFDTOTAL-FNXA200002000.htm [n/a PubMed] [90 women]

Eye (Diagnostic Value of DUS)

[YJiao2008] Yang Jiao, "Diagnostic Value of Prenatal Ultrasonography in the Fetal Eye Abnormalities", *Chinese Journal of Prenatal Diagnosis*, February 2008. http://en.cnki.com.cn/Article_en/CJFDTOTAL-ZGCQ200802009.htm [1,300 women] [n/a PubMed] [Note: This demonstrates the "Diagnostic Value" of DUS. This is, by far, the largest study within the CHS, yet it is the only study that has no control group to discount damage by stressors such as DUS.]

Immune System Dysfunction

[YGong1991] Yan Gong, Yun-Jing Zhang, and Bingsheng Wang, "Ultrasonic Influence Decidua Of Immunocompetent Cells", *Chinese Journal Of Ultrasound In Medicine*, March 1991. http://en.cnki.com.cn [n/a PubMed] [n/a subject count in Abstract]

[XHong2004] Xiao Hong, "Diagnostic Ultrasound Exposure Of Pregnant Women Late In Pregnancy Influence On Neonatal Immune Function", *Shanxi Journal of Medicine*, 2004. http://en.cnki.com.cn [n/a PubMed] [32 women]

[ZZhang1994] Zhiyou Zhang, Xiuzhen Wang, Junlan Liu, "Study On The Effect Of Newborn Erythrocyte Immune Function Exposed To Diagnostic Ultrasonic Irradiation In Pregnant Women", *Journal Of Taishan Medical College.* 1994 Feb;15(2). http://en.cnki.com.cn [n/a PubMed] [n/a subject count in Abstract]

Kidney

[ZFeng2002] Zeping Feng, "Effects of Diagnostic Ultrasonic Wave on the Ultrastructure of the Fetal Kidney of Second Trimester of Pregnancy", *Chinese Journal Of Ultrasound In Medicine*. 2002 Mar. http://en.cnki.com.cn [n/a PubMed] [18 women]

Mutagenesis

[YGong1988] Y. Gong, YJ Zhang, and BZ Wang, "An Assessment Of The Effect Of Ultrasonic Diagnostic Dosage Of The Embryos In Utero", J Ultrasound Med, Official Proceedings WFUMB Meeting (1988): 265–66. http://en.cnki.com.cn [n/a PubMed] [n/a subject count in Abstract]

[LZhang1991] Liwei Zhang, "Approach to the Mutability of Diagnostic Ultrasound", *Journal of Basic and Clinical Oncology*, February 1991. http://en.cnki.com.cn/Article_en/CJFDTOTAL-HLZL199102011.htm [n/a PubMed] [29 adults, no fetal exposure, blood SCE test, study not counted in my summary table]

Neurological

[YZhu2002] Ying-Yuan Zhu, Zi-neng Wang, Xiao-lan Shi, Xiao-Qing Luo, Fu-Xin Tang, Zu-Wen Guo, "Preliminary Study Of Effect Of Diagnostic B Ultrasound On The Ultrastructure Of Human Fetal Cerebral Neurons During Mid-Pregnancy", Journal of Jinan University, *Natural Science & Medicine*. 2002 Jun. http://en.cnki.com.cn/Article_en/CJFDTOTAL-JNDX200206016.htm [n/a PubMed] [8 women]

[YZhu2005] Ying-Yuan Zhu, X Shi, X Luo, "Effects Of Diagnostic B Ultrasound On The Ultrastructure Of Human Fetal Cerebral Neuroglia Cells During Mid-Pregnancy", *Journal Of Practical Medicine*. 2005 Mar. http://en.cnki.com.cn [n/a PubMed] [10 women]

Fetal Ovary

[ZFeng1997] Zeping Feng, Lianlian Wu, Haijun Tang, "Effects of Diagnostic Ultrasonic Wave on the Ultrastructure of Fetal Ovary of Mid-Trimester Pregnancy", *Chinese Journal Of Ultrasound In Medicine*. 1997 Dec; The Third Hospital of Changsha 410002. http://en.cnki.com.cn [n/a PubMed] [70 aborted fetuses, 120 ovaries]

[PPingze1997] Ping Pingze, "Comprehensive Studies of Diagnostic Ultrasound In Pregnancy Fetal Ovary Ultrastructure", *Chinese Journal of Ultrasound in Medicine*. 13, no. 12 (1997): 43–45. http://en.cnki.com.cn [n/a PubMed] [n/a subject count in Abstract]

Pituitary Gland Dysfunction

[ZFeng1998] Zeping Feng, Chen Hui, Lianlian Wu, "Effects of Diagnostic Ultrasonic Radiation on the Ultrastructure of Fetal Hypophysis of Mid-Trimester Gestation", *Chinese Journal Of Ultrasound In Medicine*. 1998 Nov. http://en.cnki.com.cn [28 women]

Testicles

[ZFeng1996] Zeping Feng, "Effects Of Diagnostic Ultrasonic Wave On The Ultrastructures Of The Human Fetus Testis During Midstage Pregnancy", *Chinese Journal Of Ultrasound In Medicine*. 1996 May. http://en.cnki.com.cn [n/a PubMed] [n/a subject count in Abstract]

[PPingze1996] Ping Pingze, "Comprehensive Studies of Diagnostic Ultrasound On Micro-Trimester Fetal Testis Structure", *Chinese Journal of Ultrasound in Medicine*, 12, no. 5 (1996): 12–14. http://en.cnki.com.cn [n/a PubMed] [n/a subject count in Abstract]

[HTang1995] Haijun Tang, Zeping Feng, Lianlian Wu, Hui Cheng, Yinyun Lin, Daming Tang, "Effects Of Diagnostic Ultrasonic Wave On The Ultrastructure Of Testis In Fetus",

Bulletin Of Hunan Medical University. 1995
Jun. http://en.cnki.com.cn [n/a PubMed] [16 women]

Animal Studies Conducted in China

Examples

[Author not listed], "A Review of the Advanced Studies On the Biological Effect of Diagnostic Ultrasound on Living Rats Embryos", *Journal of Practical Radiology*, June 2004.

Minli Cao, Huailu Wang, and Hongbin Zhao, "Research on the Expression of C-fos in Rat Ovary by Irradiated with Ultrasonic Wave", *Chinese Journal Of Ultrasound In Medicine*, January 2002.

Wenxui Chen, Yanqun Li, and Qin Li, "Apoptosis Induction In The Rat Oviduct Cell After Exposure To Diagnostic Ultrasound", *Chinese Journal Of Ultrasonography*, September 2002.

Zhao Jing, et al., "Effects Of Repeated Diagnostic Color Doppler Ultrasound Insonification On Protein P53 Expression And Ultrastructure Of Central Nervous System Of Fetal Rats", *Chinese Journal of Medical Imaging Technology*, August 2005.

Haitao Liu et al., "Effects of Diagnostic Ultrasound on HSP70 Expression in Chorionic Villi in Rats During Early Pregnancy and the Role of HSP70 in Apoptosis in Chorionic Villi", *International Journal of Molecular Medicine*, September 12, 2013.

Wangpen Liu, et al, "Study of Ultrasound Wave Effect on Mouse Fetus", *Chinese Journal Of Ultrasound In Medicine*, May 1996.

Suyun Meng, Ruifa Mi, and Lingling E, "Study Of The Diagnostic Ultrasound Causing Fetal Rat Brain FOS Expressing", *Chinese Journal Of Ultrasonography*, May 2000.

Suyun Meng, Zheyu Han, and Reifa Mi, "Study on Diagnostic Ultrasound Causing Inner Ear Fos Protein Expression in

Fetal Rat", *Chinese Journal Of Ultrasound In Medicine*, October 2001.

Xin Wang, Jing Huang, and Yijia Tang, "Ultrasound Induced Cell Apoptosis Following Carotid Artery Injury in Rats", *Journal of Clinical Ultrasound in Medicine*, January 2004.

Jin-jui Wang, Li-min Liu, and Jun Wei, "Comparative Study of Mouse Embryos Cells Apoptosis Induced by Variant Diagnostic Dose of Ultrasound", *Chinese Journal Of Medical Imaging Technology*, October 2003.

Jinhui Wang, Limin Liu, and Jun Wei, "Effect of Diagnostic Dose of Color Doppler Ultrasound on Mouse Embryo Cells", *Chinese Journal Of Ultrasound In Medicine*, August 2002.

Ya-Ning Wei, Jing Liu, Qing Shu, Xiao-Feng Huang, and Jing-Zao Chen, "Effects of infrasound on ultrastructure of testis cell in mice", *Zhonghua Nan Ke Xue* (*National Journal of Andrology*) 8, no. 5 (2002): 323–25, 328.

Feng-Yi Yang, et al., "Prenatal Exposure to Diagnostic Ultrasound Impacts Blood-brain Barrier Permeability in Rats", *Ultrasound in Medicine & Biology* 38, no. 6 (June 2012): 1051–57.

Zhenrong Zhang and others, "Study of Neurobehavioral Teratogenesis of Offspring of Rats Exposed to Different Ultrasound Irradiation Time on the 5th Day Gestation", *Chinese Journal Of Ultrasound In Medicine*, March 1992.

Jianpin Zhu, Jian Lin, and Baozhag Zhang, "The Mutating Effect of Color Doppler Ultrasound of Diagnostic Dosage in Rat", *Chinese Journal Of Ultrasonography*, April 1996.

Cell Studies Conducted in China

Examples

Mingsheng He, Honghua Cao, and Nianlin Zhu, "Mechanisms of K562 Cells Apoptosis Induced by Ultrasound", *Chinese Journal Of Ultrasound In Medicine*, October 2006.

Liujin Min, Jun Wei, Jingping Zhang, and Bin Wang, "B-Mode Ultrasound Study Mutagenic Effects On Root Tip Cells", *Cancer, Aberrations, Mutation Journal*, June 1996. [n/a subject count in Abstract]

Xiao-hong Xu and Luo Yi, "Effect And Mechanism Of Apoptosis Of HEK-293 Cells Induced By Diagnostic Ultrasound", *Chinese Journal of Medical Imaging Technology*, November 2008.

Luo Yi, Ran Wang, and Xiao-hong Xu, "Effect Of Ultrasound On Apoptosis Of Human Embryonic Kidney Cells", *Journal of Guangdong Medical College*, February 2010.

Tinghe Yu, Weihua Zhao, and Chunliang Zhao, "Effects of Ultrasound on Osmotic Fragility Test of Sheep Red Blood Cells", *Chinese Journal Of Ultrasound In Medicine*, December 1997.

Caixia Zhang et al., "Study of the Effect of Ultrasonic Diagnostic Dosage on Cell Growth and Cell Inhibition", *Journal of Biomedical Engineering*, March 1994.

Glossary

Acronyms

ADHD: Attention Deficit Hyperactivity Disorder, According to McClintic (2013), "Hyperactivity is so common in ASD that until recently the presence of ASD actually precluded concurrent diagnosis of ADHD."

ALARA: As Low As Reasonably Allowable (minimal DUS exposure)

ASD: Autism Spectrum Disorder, i.e., indicated by a range of neurodevelopmental disorders, such as, autism, Asperger's Syndrome, tics, personality quirks, often diagnosed in early childhood, though diagnoses can be delayed into adulthood. ADHD is officially outside this category, though ASD correlates well with ADHD.

CDC: The Center for Disease Control and Prevention, in Atlanta, Georgia.

DUS: Diagnostic ultrasound.

CHS: The Chinese Human Studies, of diagnostic ultrasound, circa 1988-2011.

MI and TI: These are displayed on DUS machine monitors. MI is "mechanical safety index" and indicates the risk of physical (mechanical) alterations of tissue. TI is "thermal safety index" and refers to risk due to rising biological temperatures via DUS exposure.

NCRPM: National Council on Radiation Protection and Measurements.

NIH: National Institutes of Health

SPTA: Spatial Peak Temporal Average. This is the standard intensity parameter for the expression of ultrasound intensity in terms of milliwatts per square centimeters, for example, 100 mW/cm2 SPTA.

Terms

Apoptosis: A natural form of "programmed cell suicide". The analogy would be leaves falling during autumn.

Arcana: Important yet buried literature, disconnected, ostracized, and herein the term refers to the CHS. The term, arcana, also refers to the similarly disconnected pesticide/polio literature of the 1940-1950s (Biskind, Mobbs, and Scobey), discovered as the result of my finalized independent research for toxicological polio causation, first published in *The Townsend Letter for Doctors and Patients*, June 2000, then widely plagiarized.

Bioeffects: Biological effects, symptoms.

B-mode: The common obstetric ultrasound machine mode.

Chorioamnion: The membranes that surround the fetus. These protect the fetus and form the maternal-fetal junction through which nutrients are transferred to the fetus.

Chorioamnionitis: Inflammation of the chorioamnion.

Conflict of interest. This can be unconscious, subconscious, interactive, and wide scale.

Critic: (Definition for this book) A person who takes the critical view, and herein, a person who argues for the inclusion of toxicology in diagnostics.

Critical study: (Definition for this book) A study that critiques the mainstream defense of environmental hazards, e.g., DUS, vaccines, EMF, etc.

Doppler Ultrasound: A type of DUS used to analyze blood flow in the cardiovascular system. Usually very high intensity. Can exceed FDA/1991 limits.

Flow cytometry: An analytic technology, utilizing lasers to count and sort cells, to detect biomarkers, and used in protein engineering. Cells and other particles are suspended in a fluid stream where they flow past an electronic detector.

Industry: Excessive and irresponsible polluting industry.

In utero: Pertaining to a study "in the uterus", where the fetus is irradiated with DUS and later analyzed, usually as birth matter following an abortion.

In vitro: Pertaining to a study "in the glass", Petri dish, test tube, etc., i.e., conducted upon tissue samples, cells, blood, etc. extracted from a living organism.

Magnitude: One order of magnitude would be in the area of a factor of 10x. Two orders of magnitude would be in the area of a factor of 100x.

Medico: A medical practitioner.

Necrosis: Death of cells due to trauma or damage from stressors such as poisoning or radiative poisoning.

Neonate: A newborn.

No Minimum Threshold: No safe dose, also called the "Linear No Threshold" model, which is generally accepted for X-Ray radiation, and arguable for DUS.

Pathogen: A disease-causing agent, nearly always a germ. This is a biased term as it generally excludes toxicological agents, even though a disease-causing agent can obviously be toxicological.

Pathologist: One who studies disease causation (biased towards germ causation).

Prenatal: Before birth, for example, with reference to a zygote or fetus.

Postnatal: That which follows birth, usually referring to a newborn child.

P-value: The probability that the observed results occurred by chance.

Ultrasound: Various terms for ultrasound are employed here, and their meaning discerned from the context. The acronym "DUS" is "diagnostic ultrasound". It can be a synonym for "obstetric ultrasound" or "prenatal ultrasound". By itself, "ultrasound" can be a synonym for DUS or a general term for the acoustic frequency range known as ultrasound.

Transducer or probe. In the context of fetal DUS, this is an ultrasound transmitter, placed directly against the mother to transmit ultrasound for the purposes of echo imaging. It usually consists of a piezoelectric crystal that oscillates commonly in the range of 2 to 9 megahertz. This is above the frequencies of the AM radio band.

Vacuoles: Chambers in cell walls or tissue, as the result of disease.

Weasel Words: Phrases that appear meaningful though conveying ambiguity to enable denial if challenged.

References and Notes

[1] Beverley Lawrence Beech, "Ultrasound: Weighing the Propaganda Against the Facts", *Midwifery Today* no. 51 (Autumn 1999)

[2] Doris Haire, "Fetal Effects of Ultrasound: A Growing Controversy*", *Journal of Nurse-Midwifery* 29, no. 4 (1984): 241–246. Note: Doris was President of American Foundation for Maternal and Child Health and Chair of Committee on Maternal and Child Health, National Women's Health Alliance in Manhattan, NY. She is deceased as of June 7, 2014. Unfortunately and coincidentally, she died during the days I was trying to contact her by email, phone, and messages hand-delivered via her concierge.

[3] Nancy Evans and Michealene Cristini Risley, "Could Prenatal Ultrasounds Contribute To Cases Of Autism?", *Huffington Post*, July 13, 2011

[4] Parrish Nelson Hirasaki, "Ultrasound Autism Connection?", www.ultrasound-autism.org

[5] Seth Roberts, "Archive For The 'Sonograms And Autism' Category", *Seth's Blog*, April 19, 2012, http://blog.sethroberts.net/category/autism/sonograms-and-autism

[6] David Blake and Rebecca Panter, "Ultrasound: Autism, Agriculture, and a Future Tool for Treating Neurological Diseases", *The University of North Carolina* (2012)

[7] Esther Thaler, "Dr Robert Mendelsohn on Pregnancy and the Dangers of Ultrasound", YouTube video, circa 1983

[8] Sarah J. Buckley, MD, "Ultrasound Scans — Cause for Concern", 2005, www.sarahbuckley.com/ultrasound-scans-cause-for-concern

[9] Robert Mendelsohn, MD, *How To Raise A Healthy Child In Spite of Your Doctor* (*Random House Publishing Group*, 1984)

[10] Marsden Wagner, "Ultrasound: More Harm than Good?", *Midwifery Today* no. 50 (*Summer* 1999)

[11] Caroline Rodgers, "Questions about Prenatal Ultrasound and the Alarming Increase in Autism", *Midwifery Today* no. 80 (Winter 2006)

[13] Jorn Olsen, Shah Ebrahim, and Chitr Sitthi-amorn, "Scientific Fraud and Epidemiology", *IEA*, June 2013

[15] The Chinese University of Hong Kong. "State Key Laboratories" www.cuhk.edu.hk/english/research/laboratory.html

[16] Caroline Rodgers, "The Elephant In The Room", 2010, archived by Parrish Nelson Hirasaki at www.ultrasound-autism.org/?page_id=522. See a slide version at IACC's website: http://iacc.hhs.gov/events/2010/slides_caroline_rodgers_102210.pdf

[17] Susan Katz Miller, "Summary: Exposure Criteria for Medical Diagnostic Ultrasound: II. Criteria Based on All Known Mechanisms", National Council on Radiation Protection and Measurements. The NCRPM document was published in 2002. Susan's document is undated but its PDF created date is 2003.

[18] David Toms, M.D., "Ultrasound Safety Inconsistency: Why Are Adult Eyes Treated with More Care than Fetal Eyes during Sonograms?", *Is Prenatal Ultrasound Safe?* www.fetalultrasoundsafety.net

[19] Mark H Ellisman, Darryl Erik Palmer, and Michael P André, "Diagnostic Levels of Ultrasound May Disrupt Myelination", *Experimental Neurology* 98, no. 1 (October 1987): 78–92

[20] Doreen Liebeskind, Robert Bases, Flora Elequin, Simon Neubort, Robin Leifer, Robert Goldberg, and Mordecai Koenigsberg, "Diagnostic Ultrasound: Effects on the DNA

and Growth Patterns of Animal Cells", *Radiology* 131, no. 1 (April 1, 1979): 177–84.

[21] Gloria LeMay "7-Step Recipe for Scrambling the Brain of a Baby", www.gloriaLeMay.com/blog/?p=247 ; Dec 2009

[22] Robert Bases of Columbia University, Letter in *Science*, 5/10/1985, Vol 228, p 650. www.sciencemag.org/content/228/4700/650.1

[23] Thomas R. Nelson, PhD, J. Brian Fowlkes, PhD, and Jacques S. Abramowicz, MD, Charles C. Church, PhD, "Ultrasound Biosafety Considerations for the Practicing Sonographer and Sonologist", *J Ultrasound Med* 28 (2009): 139–50.

[24] National Vaccine Information Center, counts vaccine doses: http://www.nvic.org/CMSTemplates/NVIC/pdf/49-Doses-PosterB.pdf

[25] Dr Carol Phillips, DC. http://www.dynamicbodybalancing.com/About_D.B.B.html

[26] Thomas R. Nelson, PhD, "Reporting of Bioeffects Research Results to the Ultrasound Community", *Journal of Ultrasound in Medicine* 24, no. 9 (September 1, 2005): 1169–70. http://www.jultrasoundmed.org/content/24/9/1169.full

[27] "Causes of Autism [7/4/2013]", *Wikipedia*, July 4, 2013. http://en.wikipedia.org/wiki/Causes_of_autism. Note: The topic of possible ultrasound causation has hence been nearly removed, including the quote by Abramowicz, "lack of... human data is appalling".

[28] Macintosh, I. J. C., and D. A. Davey, "Chromosome Aberrations Induced by an Ultrasonic Fetal Pulse Detector", *British Medical Journal* 4, no. 5727 (October 10, 1970): 92–93.

[29] "Human study" is a mainstream term, nearly always referring to population studies. These are epidemiological re-

views of clinical records, vulnerable to a chain of biased interpretations. They are actually not studies of humans, but of records made by humans. The term "human study" is semantically and politically problematic because ultrasound scientists tend not to distinguish such studies from *in utero* exposure studies. The term obfuscates the idea of *in utero* exposure studies or gives the impression that exposure studies have been done. Thus, I use the term, "*in utero* human study" to distinguish from population studies.

[30] T. A. Whittingham, "Estimated Fetal Cerebral Ultrasound Exposures from Clinical Examinations", *Ultrasound in Medicine & Biology* 27, no. 7 (July 2001): 877–82.

[31] T. A. Siddiqi, and W. D. O'Brien, Jr, "Ultrasound Exposimetry: Are Current Clinical Instruments Capable of Causing Harm to the Human Embryo or Fetus?" *ICA Sessions*, 2001. http://www.icacommission.org/Proceedings/ICA2001Rome/7_06.pdf

[32] Sarah L. Cibull, BS, Gerald R. Harris, PhD, and Diane M. Nell, PhD, "Trends in Diagnostic Ultrasound Acoustic Output From Data Reported to the US Food and Drug Administration for Device Indications That Include Fetal Applications", *J Ultrasound Med* 32 (2013): 1921–32.

[36] Z Qian, P Stoodley, and W G Pitt, "Effect of Low-Intensity Ultrasound upon Biofilm Structure from Confocal Scanning Laser Microscopy Observation", *Biomaterials* 17, no. 20 (October 1996): 1975–1980

[37] Sheiner, Eyal, Ilana Shoham-Vardi, and Jacques S. Abramowicz, "What Do Clinical Users Know Regarding Safety of Ultrasound During Pregnancy?" *Journal of Ultrasound in Medicine* 26, no. 3 (March 1, 2007): 319–25.

[38] Comparison graphs, *in situ* intensities: Ang (2006) and Ellisman (1987) provided *in situ* intensity values, measured in their laboratories. The other studies provide only device intensity values. FDA/1991 is a given *in situ* value. The AIUM Statement is a device intensity value. Where no *in situ*

value is provided, I estimated *in situ* values via the homogenous tissue attenuation protocol advocated by Siddiqi and O'Brien (2001), who conclude, "Of all the models proposed, the homogeneous tissue model is the best model for determining ultrasonic exposure risk during a reproductive ultrasonographic examination. We believe our data... can be the basis for testing for harmful biologic effects." RFeng's review concerned studies that were mostly less than 10mW/cm2 SPTA, and so I used that as an average value for his advice of 3 minutes. Dwell time: All of the mentioned critical studies are dwell time studies, i.e., no moving transducer except for RFeng's review of the CHS where clinical scenarios were often simulated. Nevertheless, I did not discount CHS dwell time, and that works greatly in favor of the industrial view, giving a much higher value for RFeng (2000) than if I were to estimate CHS dwell time.

[39] Wesley L. Nyborg, PhD, "History of the American Institute of Ultrasound in Medicine's Efforts to Keep Ultrasound Safe", J Ultrasound Med 22 (2003): 1293–1300.

[41] Professor Ruo Feng earned graduated from the University of Leningrad in the former Soviet Union, year 1961. He has won many awards, chaired many positions, and published over 180 papers re ultrasound applications ranging from obstetrics to nuclear physics. He collaborated on several major papers with T.J. Mason of Coventry University, UK.

[42] Eitan Kimmel conducts research at the Department of Biomedical Engineering, Technion Institute, in Haifa, Israel. His team has determined very low exposure thresholds for ultrasound bioeffects (symptoms ranging to irreversible damage) in animal cells. These are much lower than the exposure limits allowed by the FDA (in terms of the Mechanical Index exposure value, MI), and at much lower sound pressure levels (MPa) than generally recognized. Several of their studies have been published in *PNAS*, *Nature*, and other journals of ultrasound, radiology and engineering.

[43] D W Anderson and J T Barrett, "Ultrasound: A New Immunosuppressant", *Clinical Immunology and Immunopathology* 14, no. 1 (September 1979): 18–29

[44] A. H. Saad and A. R. Williams, "Effects of Therapeutic Ultrasound on Clearance Rate of Blood Borne Colloidal Particles in Vivo.", *The British Journal of Cancer. Supplement* 5 (March 1982): 202–205

[45] Jennifer Margulis, PhD, *The Business of Baby*, http://jennifermargulis.net/books/the-business-of-baby/

[46] Kelly Brogan, MD, "Perils of Peeking into the Womb" http://kellybroganmd.com/article/utrasound-risks-perils-of-peeking-into-the-womb/

[72] Andy Field, PhD, "Null Hypothesis Significance Testing", C8057 *(Research Methods)*, 2005

[75] Eugenius Ang, Vicko Gluncic, Alvaro Duque, Mark E. Schafer, and Pasko Rakic, "Prenatal Exposure to Ultrasound Waves Impacts Neuronal Migration in Mice", *Proceedings of the National Academy of Sciences* 103, no. 34 (August 22, 2006): 12903–10.

[77] MT Stanton et al., "Diagnostic Ultrasound Induces Change within Numbers of Cryptal Mitotic and Apoptotic Cells in Small Intestine", *Life Sciences* 68, no. 13 (February 16, 2001): 1471–1475

[80] Virtually no human studies are in the Western MM realm. I found two DUS human studies, and those are rarely mentioned

[81] Hariharan Shankar and Paul S. Pagel, "Potential Adverse Ultrasound-Related Biological Effects: A Critical Review", *Anesthesiology* 115, no. 5 (November 2011): 1109–1124

[82] Gail ter Haar, "Ultrasonic Imaging: Safety Considerations", *Interface Focus* 1, no. 4 (August 6, 2011): 686–697

[83] Melvin E. Stratmeyer et al., "Fetal Ultrasound Mechanical Effects", *Journal of Ultrasound in Medicine* 27, no. 4 (April 1, 2008): 597–605

[84] Douglas L Miller, "Safety Assurance in Obstetrical Ultrasound", *Seminars in Ultrasound, CT, and MR* 29, no. 2 (2008): 156–64.

[85] C A Kimmel, M E Stratmeyer, W D Galloway, N T Brown, J B Laborde, and H K Bates, "Developmental Exposure of Mice to Pulsed Ultrasound", *Teratology* 40, no. 4 (October 1989): 387–93.

[86] J. S. Abramowicz, "Prenatal Exposure to Ultrasound Waves: Is There a Risk?", *Ultrasound in Obstetrics and Gynecology* 29, no. 4 (2007): 363–367

[88] Jim Giles, "Ultrasound Scans Accused Of Disrupting Brain Development", *Nature* 431 (October 28, 2004): 1

[89] Susan Katz Miller, "Summary: Exposure Criteria for Medical Diagnostic Ultrasound: II. Criteria Based on All Known Mechanisms."

[90] Danica Marinac-Dabic, Cara J Krulewitch, and Roscoe M Moore Jr, "The Safety of Prenatal Ultrasound Exposure in Human Studies (FDA)", *Epidemiology (Cambridge, Mass.)* 13 Suppl 3 (May 2002): S19–22

[95] Gail ter Haar, ed., *The Safe Use Of Ultrasound In Medical Diagnosis*, 3rd ed. (The British Institute of Radiology, 2012)

[96] Y. Gong, YJ Zhang, and BZ Wang, "An Assessment Of The Effect Of Ultrasonic Diagnostic Dosage Of The Embryos In Utero", *J Ultrasound Med, Official Proceedings* WFUMB Meeting (1988): 265–266

[97] Xin-Fang Wang, "History of the Development of Ultrasound in China", www.ob-ultrasound.net/historychina.html This is Dr Joseph Woo's ultrasound website.

[103] Abbi M. McClintic, Bryan H. King, Sara J. Webb, and Pierre D. Mourad, "Mice Exposed to Diagnostic Ultrasound In Utero Are Less Social and More Active in Social Situations Relative to Controls", *International Society for Autism Research,* 7 (November 18, 2013): 295–304.

[104] K. Salvesen et al., "Safe Use of Doppler Ultrasound during the 11 to 13 + 6-Week Scan: Is It Possible?" *Ultrasound in Obstetrics & Gynecology* 37, no. 6 (2011): 628–628

[106] Kevin Martin, "The Acoustic Safety of New Ultrasound Technologies", *Ultrasound* 18, no. 3 (August 1, 2010): 110–118

[107] William D. O'Brien, Jr, PhD, John G. Abbott, PhD, et al., "Acoustic Output Upper Limits Proposition: Should Upper Limits Be Retained?", *J Ultrasound Med* no. 21 (2002): 1335–1341

[127] *Thinking Mom's Revolution* http://thinkingmomsrevolution.com

[131] Jacques S. Abramowicz, MD, "Bioeffects of Obstetric Ultrasound for the Clinician: How to Keep It Safe." October 12, 2012

[143] Ionel Rosenthal, Joe Z Sostaric, and Peter Riesz, "Sonodynamic Therapy--a Review of the Synergistic Effects of Drugs and Ultrasound." *Ultrasonics Sonochemistry* 11, no. 6 (September 2004): 349–63

[147] A. Cardinale et al., "Bioeffects of Ultrasound: An Experimental Study on Human Embryos", *Ultrasonics* 29, no. 3 (May 1991): 261–263

[162] William D. O'Brien, Edwin L. Carstensen, and Wesley L. Nyborg, "Acoustic Society Award 1998: Floyd Dunn", http://acousticalsociety.org/about/awards/gold/12_10_10_dunn. Accessed 12/22/2013

[170] Glaxo Pharmaceuticals, Flulaval brand flu vaccine, product description: www.harvoa.org/polio/flu/glaxo-ins.htm

[172] No Spray Coalition, Mitchel Cohen, Coordinator, www.nospray.org

[173] "Home Birth - Wikipedia", Wikipedia, the Free Encyclopedia, February 9, 2015. http://en.wikipedia.org/w/index.php?title=Home_birth

[174] C. Seife, "Research Misconduct Identified by the US Food and Drug Administration: Out of Sight, Out of Mind, Out of the Peer-Reviewed Literature", *JAMA Intern Med.*, February 9, 2014.

[175] Jacques S. Abramowicz, Peter A. Lewin, and Barry B. Goldberg, "Ultrasound Bioeffects for the Perinatologist", In *The Global Library of Women's Medicine*, updated 2011.

[176] Christof Sohn, Klaus Vetter, and Hans-Joachim Voigt. Doppler *Ultrasound in Gynecology and Obstetrics*. Thieme, 2011.

[177] Kenneth Rock and Hajime Kono, "The Inflammatory Response to Cell Death", *Annual Review of Pathology* 3 (2008): 99–126.

[178] Roche Applied Science. "Apoptosis, Cell Death, and Cell Proliferation Manual. 3rd edition."

The Author

Jim West was raised in Arizona where he was fortunate to have experienced beautiful deserts, mountains and sky-scapes. He attended Arizona State University with a double major in mechanical engineering and music composition. He is autodidact in virology, toxicology, organic chemistry, electronics, and ultrasound.

After three years in the U.S. military, Jim moved to New York City, where he became involved in computer consultancy, environmental research, politics, and the arts. He served as Chairman of the Science Committee for the No Spray Coalition, which litigated extensively against the City of New York with regard to the helicopter pesticide spray programs that began circa 1999. He is a member of Greenspeakers, a Toastmasters group, and a member of the Advisory Board of Discovery Salud.

Jim is known for his published articles describing independent discoveries of environmental causation for polio, West Nile, SARS, and H1N1 epidemics. In 2001, Nicholas Regush, producer and journalist for ABC, wrote a lengthy article, "West Nile: Virus or Environment?", describing Jim's findings that unpublicized MTBE petrochemical air pollution had been severely increasing air pollution levels in the New York City region. The article was very well received by the ABC News online readership. Regush several times spoke of the possibility of bringing Jim's work to ABC's evening shows such as *20/20* and *Nightline*, with ABC's "top brass" interested in Jim's work, however, Jim was wary of such intense publicity.

Books by Jim West

Ultrasound Causation for Microcephaly and Zika Virus
The Hypothesis (Part A)
Published 10/2017.

Ultrasound Causation for Microcephaly and Zika Virus
The Hypothesis (Part B)
See www.harvoa.org for availability.

Ultrasound Causation for Microcephaly and Zika Virus
The Hypothesis (Part C)
See www.harvoa.org for availability.

50 Human Studies: A New Bibliography
[This book on ultrasound]
Published 5/2015

DDT/Polio
Published 2013

Copyright

Brief passages and two images may
be copied without permission,
providing that Jim West and www.harvoa.org
are clearly referenced.

Please credit Jim West for
his research and bibliographical compilations.

Contact:
www.harvoa.org/contact

71005074R00083

Made in the USA
Columbia, SC
24 August 2019